A Diet
for
All Reasons

A Diet For All Reasons

Nutrition Guide & Recipe Collection

Paulette Eisen

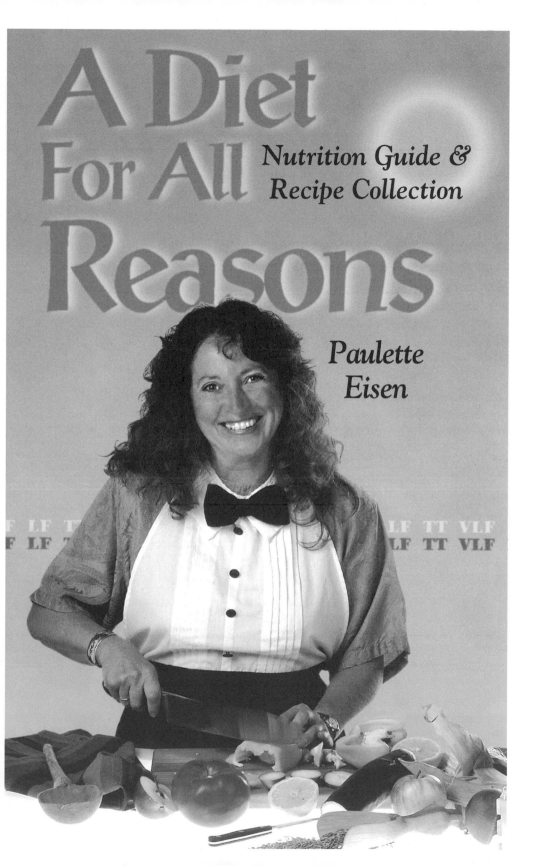

Published by:

Alive Books
PO Box 80055
Burnaby BC Canada V5H 3X1

Cover Design & Typesetting: Peter Virag
Front & Back Cover Photos: Ron Crompton

First Printing: October 1995

Canadian Cataloguing in Publication Data

Eisen, Paulette.
  A diet for all reasons

  ISBN 0-920470-68-8

  1. Vegetarianism. 2. Vegetarian cookery I. Title.
TX392.E37 1995   613.2'62   C95-911022-4

Printed and bound in Canada

*To my son Adam,
and to all other vegetarians,
past, present and future,
who have promoted and continue
to promote a health-enhancing diet,
not only for the sake of humans,
but also for all life
on this planet*

Recipe Codes

TT   – *Tasty Transition*

LF   – *Low Fat*

VLF – *Very Low Fat*

Table of Contents

Part I.   Nutrition Guide

Part II.   Recipe Collection

Foreword

As a physician and nutrition educator, writing a foreword to this recipe collection is the fulfillment of a dream. To know that every recipe that follows is free of cholesterol, low in fat and sodium and filled with foods that will enhance the health of those who partake of them, fills me with pride and satisfaction. These recipes have been developed, collected and assembled with great love and care by Ms. Paulette Eisen and then prepared to verify that they are not only healthy for the body, but also pleasing to the taste. Preparing and enjoying these foods will take you on a journey of education as well as health, and the guidelines given in these pages make the transition to cholesterol-free eating easy, nutritious and fun. You will encounter some ingredients and dishes that will probably be new to you but we hope many of them will soon become preferred favorites – and then "old friends", looked forward to with great anticipation and delight.

We hope that as you understand the principles of cholesterol-free foods you will be encouraged to explore and create your own variations. These recipes are gifts, from our hearts to yours, and with them go our most sincere wishes that the foods they bring to you will become part of the foundation of the best era of your life – one filled with health, happiness, joy and peace. Enjoy!

Michael Klaper M.D.

Michael Klaper, MD

Acknowledgements

My sincere thanks to all who gave generously of their ideas and recipes for this collection.

Marilyn Diamond whose book *The American Vegetarian Cookbook* is a classic.

Jennifer Raymond whose delicious recipes are from her wonderful book *The Peaceful Palate*.

Debra Wasserman from her book *Simply Vegan*, that supplied me with great quick and easy recipes.

Meredith McCarthy, the most meticulous cookbook writer that I have ever met, gave me some foolproof recipes from her two popular cookbooks entitled, *American Macrobiotic Cuisine* and *Fresh from a Vegetarian Kitchen*.

Cynthia Holzapfel from The Book Publishing Company supplied me with an assortment of cookbooks, including:

The Tempeh Cookbook by Dorothy Bates
Tofu Cookery by Louise Hagler
Tofu Quick and Easy by Louise Hagler
The Now and Zen Epicure by Miyoko Nashimoto
Vegetarian Cooking for Diabetics by Patricia Mozzer

Sandra Belgrade and Patricia Sweeney-Park have written a delightfully creative cookbook entitled, *Guess Who's Coming to Dinner*, with the traditional recipe on one side and its transformed, more healthful counterpart on the other.

Lynn Gale, PhD of the Vegetarian Foundation for her tips and suggestions.

My thanks to the wonderful pioneering chefs from The Vegan Restaurant in Maui and to my friend and fellow cooking instructor, Tatiania Wrenfeather and her sister, Gené Stephenson.

A special thank you to Michael James, RD who kindly donated his time to analyze the recipes in this collection.

My thanks to Alan Ross for his encouragement.

And finally my deep appreciation for my friend, my medical and nutrition advisor, Dr. Michael Klaper for his tireless devotion to seek out Truth and share it with others. Without his help, this book would not have been possible, especially the information and ideas in the transition guide, to which he made a significant contribution.

Paulette Eisen

Paulette Eisen
October, 1995

A Personal Introduction

What romance novels or detective stories are to some, cookbooks are to me: escape into adventure, romance and excitement. The difference is that I can go into my kitchen and bring these fantasies to life!

I love to read recipe books and, unlike other passions that grow weak with time, this one remains as strong as ever. I am delighted that low-fat, high fiber, natural food cuisine continues to evolve with more and more excellent chefs who are converting standard recipes and creating wonderful new recipes that couple nutrition with good taste.

Times have certainly changed since twenty years ago when I began teaching healthy wholefood cooking in British Columbia, Canada. I used to show my students how to make their own tofu because the only place we could purchase it was Chinatown. Today, tofu is sold everywhere, from natural food stores to supermarkets. Thank goodness that ingredients and equipment are readily available to today's health-minded cooks.

In 1990, I began a professional association with Dr. Michael Klaper, who was my longtime friend and doctor. We both had become aware that we had a similar vision. We both wanted to promote the benefits of a plant-based diet, high in fiber, complex carbohydrates, vitamins and minerals. Based on our personal and professional experiences and the scientific literature, we knew that this information could have far reaching effects in the treatment and prevention of disease, the health of the environment, and in the lives of countless farm animals. I saw this objective as a win/win on every level and still do.

In order to reach a larger population, beyond those who attended my or Dr. Klaper's presentations, we took two steps. One was to establish a non-profit organization, known as the Institute of Nutrition Education, whose main purpose was to educate health professionals about the strong link between diet and disease. The other was to develop and promote a multi-media program, now known as *A Diet for All Reasons*, to provide people with the information and the tools to make either a gradual or swift change to a plant-based diet. The first product to become available was a video of Dr. Klaper giving a dynamic presentation on nutrition. This was later followed by this transition guide and recipe book, and a seven-audiotape Wellness Series on the following topics: arthritis, osteoporosis, cancer, clogged arteries, weight loss, allergies and autoimmune conditions, pregnancy and children, sex and impotence, exercise, stress and diabetes. Dr. Klaper describes these conditions in his clear, easy to understand manner, and then discusses the nutritional component in terms of prevention and treatment.

For many people who had seen and been inspired by the video, *A Diet for All Reasons*, or by Dr. Klaper's lectures, the practical application of his recommendations seemed daunting. Many working women in particular, whose role it was to purchase and prepare food for their family members did not enjoy the meals. Still others who ate out a lot were worried about what they could eat in a restaurant.

I developed this book with all these factors in mind, especially as I also have shared the same concerns. Having grown up in a family in which both parents were professional cooks, our enjoyment of food was a major focal point. In the recipes in this book, taste and speed of preparation are considerations equally important as nutritional content. The transition section is full of ideas and hints about how to shop and set up your kitchen, and how to deal with all situations that involve food.

The recipes reflect years of reading, testing and teaching. The wonderful and gifted cooks who developed some of them transform nutritional principles into delicious meals for you and your family. Many have written cookbooks that I highly recommend because the recipes are consistently good throughout. In this collection, some recipes in this collection have been modified to lower fat versions. Each recipe is marked with either VLF – very low fat, LF – low fat, or TT – tasty transition with about 30% fat content.

In this new edition of my book, I have added more of my own recipes as well as a section on making the transition to a health supporting diet. Whatever choices you make regarding the food you eat, whether you adopt a completely vegan diet or elect to include more vegan meals in your food plan, I hope that this book and the other *A Diet for all Reasons* products are of help to you and those you love.

I welcome your comments or suggestions, at:

1824 Hillhurst Avenue
Los Angelos CA 90027
Tel: 310-289-4173

Part I

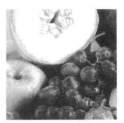

Nutrition Guide

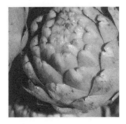

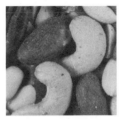

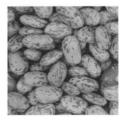

Chapter One

~ Toward a Healthy Diet

The Bad News ...

Over time, eating a high-fat, low-fiber diet based on meats, dairy and other animal products will result in a major portion of the population suffering from obesity, clogged arteries, high blood pressure and damaged hearts.

The Good News....

Fortunately, in the 1990s we have learned the lessons of our recently industrialized past, and we now know the wise steps that anyone can take to increase his/her chances for a long disease-free life.

While many formulas have been advanced over the years, scientific studies have identified seven elements that are essential for creating a healthy, energetic body. A day that includes the following is a healthy day.

1. Feed your body a "clean-burning" fuel, one that keeps the arteries free-flowing and brings oxygen-rich blood to the tissues.

This means a cholesterol-free wholefood diet. In other words, the less animal fat, cholesterol and processed foods you run through your bloodstream, and the more whole grains, fresh fruits and vegetables, and legumes you eat, the healthier you are going to be.

2. Take your body out for a good walk or some other form of exercise and stretch your joints and muscles well at least every other day.

3. Get sufficient sleep every night (preferably with the window open) or nap during the day.

4. Drink plenty of water, including a glass of fresh vegetable or fruit juice in the morning and a glass or two of pure water between every meal.

5. Get a reasonable amount of sunshine: ten to fifteen minutes of early morning or late afternoon sun.

6. Breathe deeply to oxygenate your blood and to relieve stress.

7. Get as much love and happiness flowing through your life as you can by continuing to learn and grow, and by doing for others. Love yourself as much as you would want to be loved. Laugh a lot and hug a lot.

The purpose of this book is to focus on the first element – a health-enhancing diet based on whole natural foods, low in saturated fat and cholesterol free.

Leading Experts Agree

Many experts agree with Dr. Mark Hegsted, a nutritional scientist from Harvard University, who testified before the Federal Trade Commission and stated: "I think it is clear that the American diet is indicated as a cause of coronary heart disease. And, it is pertinent, I think, to point out that the same diet is now found guilty in terms of many forms of cancer: breast cancer, cancer of the colon and others ..."

According to the Director of the Institute for Nutrition Education and Research, Michael Klaper MD, from his video and audio tapes titled *A Diet for all Reasons*, these are the health improvements you can expect when you switch from a meat based to a health-enhancing, plant-based diet.

Arteries clogged with cholesterol and atherosclerotic build-up begin to open up, leading to improvement (and often complete resolution!) of artery disorders like high blood pressure, angina pectoris or clogged leg arteries.

Sore, arthritic joints often become less painful or even pain-free.

If impotence due to atherosclerosis has been a problem, sexual potency can return, often surprisingly quickly, as arteries open.

Nasal congestion and post-nasal drip frequently clears as allergy-inciting dairy protein is eliminated from the diet

Skin rashes and eczemas frequently subside.

Headaches, including migraines, often improve or cease.

Asthma often markedly improves, or disappears altogether, as dairy products and other offending substances leave the diet.

Heartburn and indigestion predictably diminish as concentrated meat proteins that induce large acidic responses in the stomach are omitted.

Heavy menstrual flow often becomes lighter (as the intake of fatty foods that raise female hormone [estrogen] levels is reduced) thus lessening the risk for iron-deficiency anemia.

Premenstrual Syndrome (PMS) often noticeably improves or goes away altogether.

Constipation can be expected to clear quickly due to the fiber content of whole grains and vegetables.

Through your transition to better health, you can also expect to:

Learn many new and wonderful things about your body, and the foods that make you feel your best,

Taste and enjoy new and delicious foods, and

Meet other health-minded, energetic people as the world of nutritious eating opens to you.

Congratulations! You are being good to yourself and saying YES to life!

Note: see Resource section for more information on the full range of *A Diet for All Reasons* products.

Power Foods and Vital Foods

Dr. Klaper has said many times that, contrary to popular belief, the human body has absolutely no requirements for the flesh of animals or the milk of cows and in fact, runs superbly on a diet with little or no products of animal origin. Since the beginning of history humans have thrived on foods primarily grown from the earth and do so by the hundreds of millions around the world today. Food choices free of meat and dairy products are not only free of the hormones, antibiotics and other contaminants so frequently found in animal-based foods, but lower the risk of clogged arteries, high blood pressure, osteoporosis and many forms of cancer and are the basis for a wise food-choice strategy for the 1990s.

Fortunately markedly reducing and even eliminating animal products from the diet is not only health-enhancing and economical but also it is also nutritionally sound.

All the protein, vitamins, minerals and other nutrients you need are readily available from cholesterol-free grains, potatoes, fruits, vegetables and other plant-based foods.

Medical studies confirm that people who do not consume meats or dairy products and who eat a broad variety of plant-based foods are not only fully nourished, but live longer and are freer of degenerative conditions such as high blood pressure, elevated cholesterol levels and osteoporosis. Recommended reading: *McDougall's Medicine: A Challenging Second Opinion.*

Power Foods

Most of your meals should center on a dense, satisfying, carbohydrate-rich "Power Food", namely potatoes or whole grains (rice, corn, wheat, oats, barley, millet, etc.). Lest you fear that such foods are bland or coarse, realize that there are many tasty and familiar forms in which to enjoy these Power Foods – namely, in pastas, breads, cereals, casseroles, thick soups and stews and in many delightful ethnic dishes from international cuisines. Because of their low-fat nature yet high content of fiber and other complex carbohydrates, you can eat your fill of these whole foods and still watch your body become leaner and healthier.

Legumes (any food that grows in a pod, like beans, peas, chickpeas and lentils) as well as nuts and seeds are also dense Power Foods, but because of their concentrated protein and oils, you should limit your intake: legumes – one cup per day and nuts and seeds – ½ cup. Legumes can be added to soups, stews, casseroles and many other dishes.

Have at least six to eleven servings of Power Foods each day. A serving contains about five grams of protein and fifty to one hundred calories. In real life terms, a Power Food serving can be thought of as: a slice of bread, a cup of rice, a large potato or a bowl of cereal.

Vital Foods

The foods that contain the vitamins and minerals that are necessary to "burn" the energy stored in the Power Foods are the "living foods": fresh green and yellow vegetables and fresh fruits. We refer to these as "Vital Foods." The more vivid and colorful the vegetable or fruit flesh the higher its content of nutrients. A serving of Vital Food is a piece of fruit (like a banana, an apple, a peach or a glass of cool fruit smoothie), or a whole vegetable (like an ear of corn, a medium tomato or a half cup of steamed greens) or a helping of salad.

You need five to nine servings of Vital Foods each day. Try to have at least two servings of Vital Foods with every meal plus a Vital Food snack or two during the day or evening.

A healthful guideline, at least initially, is to have half your daily food intake as Power Foods and half as fresh Vital Foods. At certain times, you may want to eat proportionately more Vital Foods or Power Foods.

IMPORTANT: If you have special nutritional needs such as: pregnancy, healing an illness or raising a growing child, listen to the specific tapes in A *Diet for all Reasons* audio Wellness Series that address these issues.

The more you incorporate these Power Foods and Vital Foods into your diet the sooner you will find that choosing healthy foods becomes second nature, while unhealthy foods will become increasingly unappetizing.

Foods in the Health-Enhancing Diet

Power Foods
(6-11 daily servings)
Whole grains, nuts
Potatoes
Legumes
Products made from the above

Vital Foods
(5-9 daily servings)
Fresh green vegetables and seeds
Fresh yellow vegetables
Fresh fruits
Products made from the above

A well-balanced daily food intake might look something like the "Daily Intake Example" shown below.

Vital Foods / Power Foods: Daily Intake Example

Breakfast
1 cup cereal with ½ cup soy milk topped with
1 cup sliced strawberries and peaches plus
2 slices of whole grain toast spread with
1 T almond butter
1 small glass of fresh apple juice

Lunch
1 cup hearty vegetable soup
1 serving of tossed green salad plus
hearty sandwich consisting of
2 slices of whole grain bread with
lettuce, sprouts and tomatoes, spread with
2 T of chick pea spread (hummus)

Dinner
An Italian-style meal, with:
2 servings of spaghetti topped with
1 cup tomato and mushroom sauce
For side dishes:
1 cup steamed carrots
1 cup steamed broccoli
1 glass of sparkling mineral water mixed with fruit juice

Dessert
1 serving of apple crisp

Snacks during day
Banana

Characteristics of Health-Enhancing Foods

Cholesterol free. You do not need to supplement your diet with cholesterol since your body produces all that it needs. In fact, the best way to let the cholesterol in your blood find its own safe level is to eat a cholesterol-free diet.

Low-fat. Keep your average daily fat intake to about 20% of your total calorie intake unless you are overweight, have clogged arteries, cancer or diabetes, in which case no more than 10% is recommended.

Moderate in protein: less than 60 grams per day. (A slice of whole grain bread has about 5 grams of protein.) Remember, where protein is concerned more is not better. Most Americans eat over 100 grams of protein daily with damaging effects throughout their body. Plant protein is less concentrated than animal-based protein and thus is far safer for bones and kidneys. ("Osteoporosis" from *A Diet for All Reasons* audio Wellness Series)

High fiber and complex carbohydrates for healthy bowel and colon function lowers your risk of colon cancer.

High in antioxidants, the beta-carotene and vitamins C and E found in fresh fruits and vegetables help to protect you against cancer and premature aging.

Whole and as unprocessed and fresh as possible: if it comes in a box, bag or can, chances are the food product is processed and missing essential fiber. Whole and unprocessed foods include whole, fresh vegetables, fruits and grains.

Using Oils

Excessive amounts of oils can impede blood flow through small blood vessels, contribute to obesity and, some believe, raise your risk for some cancers. Since there are naturally occurring oils (which your body needs) in grains, nuts and seeds, cooking with oils is kept to a minimum in this book. If you are going to cook with oils, be sure to use unrefined, expeller-pressed oils such as olive or almond.

It is recommended that you have a teaspoon to a tablespoon a day of fresh pressed, unrefined oil such as flaxseed, sesame or pumpkin as these contain essential fatty acids.

Important Food Guidelines

Once you begin your transition to a health-enhancing diet keep in mind these important guidelines.

Fruit sugars can raise triglyceride levels. If you have elevated triglyceride levels, restrict your fruit consumption to less than three servings a day and your fresh fruit juice consumption to 1 small glass per day until your body has restored its triglycerides to safe levels. For Vital Foods have more fresh vegetables rather than sweet fruits.

Assure sufficient vitamin B-12 consumption by eating B-12 fortified cereals, breads or other products (nutritional yeast, soy milk, etc: read the labels) or taking a B-12 vitamin supplement (such as Super Blue-Green Algae) at least three times a week.

Substances Your Body Does Not Need

You are already familiar with the Power Foods and Vital Foods your body needs. Now, let us think about eliminating harmful substances that your body surely does not need to be healthy.

Sugar: Refined sugars can put your blood sugar on a roller coaster and leave you craving food, fatigued or gaining unwanted weight. Packaged cereals, sweetened fruit drinks, desserts and soft drinks contain a tremendous amount of sugar (eg. up to fifteen teaspoons in a can of cola). If you want sweets go for the natural ones contained in whole fruits and fresh fruit juices.

Salt: Excessive salt can contribute to raising your blood pressure, but a pinch for flavoring is acceptable. However if you are a "salt sensitive" person with high blood pressure, be aware that large amounts of soy sauces have an excessive amount of salt. If you have high blood pressure you can purchase low-sodium versions of these products.

Caffeine: Caffeine can raise your blood cholesterol and drain calcium from your bones by increasing the amount lost through the urine by the kidneys. Minimize your caffeine intake or better yet, avoid it altogether. There are many excellent coffee-like beverage alternatives such as Pero, Roma, Postum, and Cafix that many people tend to prefer once they've tried them. These products are grain-based and caffeine-free and are readily available at most natural food stores.

Alcohol: In addition to being a calcium thief and causing excretion of calcium through the urine, alcohol is a toxin to every tissue in the body especially the brain, heart, muscles, nerves, pancreas and liver. Minimize its use (one to two glasses of wine per day) or better yet, avoid it.

The Transition Plan

"If we do not change the direction in which we're going, we'll end up where we're heading ..." – Old Chinese Proverb

To help you move in the direction of a starch-based, cholesterol-free, whole food diet as quickly and conveniently as possible, a five-step Transition Plan has been designed to meet the needs of various types of individuals.

The Gradual Transition

If you are making a gradual transition, the rate at which you move through the steps of the Transition Plan is less important than the fact that you keep moving. Take as much time as you need with any given step until you are truly ready to move to the next one.

Some people take a few weeks to become comfortable with automatically choosing healthier foods, some take a few months, some take a few (or even many) years.

All of these progressions are completely acceptable because they reflect the way that people actually change their diets. In fact, you are bound to be more successful in your efforts when you are authentic and realistic with yourself. It is only when you try to change out of guilt or "because you should" that you start to experience resentment, frustration and, ultimately, a lack of progress. The most important thing is that you keep progressing toward better health.

The Rapid Transition

Some people move immediately to a health-enhancing diet and never look back. These are highly-motivated people who either have recently received a serious medical diagnosis and know that rapid dietary changes are imperative or they are people who have strong beliefs (about the environment or ethics) that compel them to change to healthier eating patterns as rapidly as possible.

If you have a serious medical problem such as an elevated cholesterol level (total over 180 mg/dl or HDL under 35 mg/dl) or high blood pressure (over 150/90 mm/Hg or 4.4 mmol/dl) and are under a physician's care for diabetes or any other serious medical condition, you are advised to make a rapid transition to healthier eating by instituting all five of the Transition Plan steps at once.

Consult with your physician to confirm that you do not have a medical condition that would prevent you from adopting a low-fat, high-fiber diet and regular exercise program. Then monitor your progress together so that you can reduce your medications as your needs for them decrease.

Individuals with Increased Calorie Needs

If you are a growing child, a pregnant woman, a healthy person who wants to gain weight or a healthy worker or athlete with significant physical demands, you will need to include more foods with higher fat and calorie content in your diet. The recipe section contains numerous Tasty Transition (TT) recipes designed with these types of individuals in mind and at least one or two helpings of these more calorie-dense style meals each day should supply the needed extra nutrients. "Rich" but cholesterol-free foods like nut butters (almond, cashew, etc.), bean spreads, tofu-based gravies and dressings are your friends. Enjoy them all without guilt and witness the positive effect.

The Five-Step Transition Plan

You will find that the following five steps become easier, even second nature, as you learn to prepare health-enhancing foods and begin to enjoy eating them regularly. Taste preferences are learned and your palate and tongue will re-educate themselves in a surprisingly short time. You can progress through these steps over several weeks or months (gradual transition) or all at once (rapid transition).

Step One: Choose fat-free versions of dairy products; eliminate egg yolks.

Choose fat-free dairy products over high-fat dairy products – this step alone will produce a major reduction in your daily fat intake.

Reduce or eliminate egg yolks by using egg substitutes.

Replace white sugar, white flour and other refined carbohydrates with whole grain-products and natural fruit-derived sweeteners. (See the Smart Shopping section)

When you have mastered step one above, move on to the next step:

Step Two: Exchange red meat for health-supporting grain, legume and potato-based dishes.

On an ever-more frequent basis replace red meat entrées with protein-rich grains and legume-based dishes such as bean burritos, tofu burgers, potato-lentil soup and bread. Do not worry, you will get all the high-quality protein you need from the Power Foods you eat.

Start by serving yourself larger and larger portions of rice, potatoes and vegetables at meals and smaller portions of meat. When you want second helpings make sure you take seconds of the rice and potatoes, not the meat. Eat your fill of these cholesterol-free foods. No feelings of deprivation allowed!

Step Three: Utilize vegetables, nuts and other protein-rich, cholesterol-free foods in exchange for poultry and fish.

When you phase red meat out of your diet you can find yourself as a poultry-and-fish eater, a stage that many people are in these days. It is important to realize, however, that chicken and fish are not health foods. They still have a very high fat content when compared to plant-based foods and they raise cholesterol levels in your blood and contribute to obesity as much as red meats.

They also tend to contain dangerous contaminants. For example, chickens are known to regularly contain toxic salmonella bacteria. While fish are the most contaminated of the flesh foods because of their exposure to pollutants such as sewage, industrial toxins and pesticides which end up in our water supply. So, when the time feels right begin to replace these flesh foods with more wholesome ones – and we advise sooner rather than later.

Begin to reduce the proportions of the chicken and fish that you use in recipes and substitute more vegetables, mushrooms, nuts, seeds and other concentrated foods.

For example, if you are making stir-fried vegetables with chicken over rice increase the amount of vegetables you use and especially add protein-rich foods such as mushrooms, tofu chunks and nuts (like almonds or cashews), while decreasing the amount of poultry used. Soon you will leave out the poultry altogether and be healthier for it. Grilled tofu cutlets substitute nicely for fish fillets and are free of cholesterol and today's ocean contaminants.

Step Four: Exchange simple, non-dairy foods for the low-fat dairy products.

Now you can eliminate the low-fat dairy products from your diet. This is an important move as it eliminates many health-endangering dairy proteins that can cause many people to suffer low-grade allergic problems such as chronically stuffed noses, constipation, congested sinuses and post-nasal drip.

The Recipe Collection, as well as the refrigerator case at the local natural food store, has many ideas for non-dairy products to take the place of milk, cream cheese, sour cream, ice cream and other dairy products.

At this time it is important to increase your consumption of calcium-rich dark leafy greens, (especially broccoli, kale, mustard greens and chard) carrots and fresh juices made from these vegetables, as well as calcium fortified orange juice, soy milk and tofu.

Step Five: Reduce or replace the "luxury fats".

Hydrogenated oils are artificially thickened vegetable oils that can damage artery walls.

Eliminate hydrogenated vegetable oils from your diet and minimize oil altogether. As a substitute for cooking oils try cooking in broth or sautéing in water.

Implementing the Transition Plan

To implement these beneficial changes in your daily diet try the following strategy.

Learn to prepare at least one cholesterol-free breakfast and then increase it to two or three. (See the "Breakfasts" chapter and listen to the accompanying audio tape for many delicious ideas.) Begin to have these wholesome breakfasts more frequently during the week until at least five out of seven breakfasts are cholesterol-free.

At the same time, prepare a cholesterol-free dinner at least once a week. Be sure to make enough to eat the next day for lunch. Begin to have these cholesterol-free lunches and dinners more frequently during the week until at least five out of seven meals are cholesterol-free.

Be sure to have a fresh Vital Food at each meal, such as fresh fruits or fruit juices, a mixed green salad, fresh or steamed greens.

Other guidelines for the journey to better health are as follows.

1. *Lower your saturated fat and cholesterol intake by choosing cholesterol-free fruits, vegetables and whole grain products over animal-based and processed foods whenever possible.*

2. *Eat more foods in their uncooked or lightly steamed state.*

3. *Purchase a good juicer and begin to drink fresh juices from fruits and vegetables at least once daily. (Optional)*

4. *Obtain a source of pure water for all your food preparation and drinking purposes.*

The Importance of a Supportive Environment

We have tried to make your transition to healthy eating as easy and smooth as possible. However, it would be misleading not to acknowledge that the journey away from the old and familiar may be extremely challenging at times.

Sharing Your Commitment with Family

An important part of making a smoother transition to a healthier lifestyle is to establish healthy relationships and to surround yourself with family and friends who will encourage you on your path to better health. Discuss your Transition Plan with your family members and enlist their help. Let them lovingly know that you are not going to insist that your food choices become theirs but you are going to want them to respect your new commitment to better health. Explain that they may try as little or as much as they like of your health-supporting foods. Watch how their comments change as they find out how good these foods taste!

Finding Like-Minded Friends

An empowering move is to start your own "support group" with health-minded friends. A good place to find these new friends is at clubs or events that are advertised at your local natural food store. A very effective, not to mention fun, method is to arrange weekly potlucks and bring a cholesterol-free dish to share – with recipes. Plan restaurant outings with friends and family. Begin trading recipes with health-minded friends, along with books, videos, and audio tapes. Shop together, clean out your kitchens and cupboards together, and talk about your challenges and new ideas. These activities go a long way towards reinforcing your new understandings and tastes, and keep you moving on the path of good eating. You will find the whole process easier and much more enjoyable.

To increase your confidence, your resolve and your appreciation for the style of eating the Transition Plan introduces you to, become educated and aware of the vast scope of books, tapes and other materials that are available on the subject of natural foods, improved health through nutrition and global ecology. To start check the recommended reading list in the back of this book.

What to Do When You Want That Cheeseburger?

I suggest that you think about it first and how it will affect you and if you still want it go ahead and eat it. Many report that once they have made the transition to a meat-free diet, that having a cheeseburger results in deeply felt body discomfort and is motivation enough not to repeat it.

Chapter Two

~Breakfasts

The Purpose of a Good Breakfast

Why have a good breakfast? For a very simple reason – it is the beginning of your day. Put your best foot forward.

A good breakfast should get you off to the right nutritional start each day – supplying your energy needs without leaving you either sleepy or famished by mid-morning. Only you can determine the right breakfast for you. Since your body changes over time and with the seasons you will probably want to vary your breakfast patterns. Your body knows best – listen to it and eat what makes you feel the best.

For example, you may prefer a light breakfast during the hot summer months, and a denser one during the cold winter. Or you may prefer to fix a quick breakfast during the week while spending more time in the kitchen over the week end.

Quick Start Breakfast Ideas

If your primary criteria for breakfast is quick and nutritious, then mix and match the following breakfast ideas.

Fruit juice: preferably freshly juiced

Fresh fruit: such as a ½ grapefruit or ½ cantaloupe

Fruit bowl: cut up your favorite fruits and top them with fruit juice. Have plenty if you wish.

Smoothies: use a base of fresh apple juice and frozen or fresh bananas. Add frozen berries or other fruits. If desired add whole food supplements such as Super Blue-Green Algae. Add cantaloupe, cut into chunks and blended on high speed. That's all. You'll love it and it is so nutritious!

Miso Soup: with or without rice, noodles and vegetables. Nice and warming on a cold morning.

Dry whole grain cereals: without added sugar, fats, preservatives or additives, served with fruit and topped with fruit juice or non-dairy milks (see below).

Granola: (oil-free),topped with fruit or mixed with applesauce or soy yogurt.

Hot cereal: like oatmeal, or Cream of Rye from Roman Meal. Top with cinnamon, raisins or fruit and serve with non-dairy milks or a little maple syrup.

Whole grain toast or bagels: with fruit conserves or rice cake with apple butter.

Sprouted wheat or Essene breads: found in the refrigerator section of your neighborhood health food store, are naturally sweet without added fat or sweetener.

Fat-free muffins: either ones you have made yourself, or from Health Valley.

Leftover rice mixed with cinnamon, raisins and maple syrup.

Banana blended with ½ cup of water makes a "milk" you can use with cereal or cooked grains.

Almond butter spread on apple slices is a favorite for children and is also a great snack.

If you have slightly more time in the morning try the following: (See recipe collection for delicious and nutritious variations of these basics.)

Pancakes or waffles with syrup

Potatoes, hash browns, baked, oven fries

Scrambled tofu

French toast.

Dairy Alternatives

At breakfast, when you are deciding what to pour on your cereal remember that there are other cool sweet liquids that you can use besides cow's milk. Examples of the non-dairy milks are described below.

See Milks and Creams in Recipe Section. The secret to these recipes is to own a good blender and to use very cold water. With a little practice, a pitcher of sweet, white, frothy "milk" can be ready for drinking or pouring on fruit or cereal in five minutes.

For a change try pouring apple or other fruit juice on your cereal. Fruit juices are cold and sweet and especially convenient while traveling.

Commercial soy milk preparations like Edensoy, Westsoy-Lite, and Vitasoy keep well and are delicious for drinking. Liquid and powdered soy milks are available at your natural food store. Soyagen and Soyamel are fortified with calcium, protein, riboflavin, B-12, and Vitamin D. Note: Do not use these beverages as infant formulas. There are specially constituted formulas for this purpose.

Rice Dream, a milk made from rice, is an excellent alternative and low in fat.

Westbrae-Lite non-dairy creamer, available at natural food stores can be used with coffee or a coffee substitute such as Roma or Cafix, healthier than a caffeine fix.

Margarine Is NOT an Alternative

Contrary to popular belief, margarine is not an acceptable alternative to the high saturated fat and cholesterol of butter. This is because margarine contains hydrogenated vegetable oils that act like saturated fat in your body and can raise your cholesterol levels and thus lead to artery damage. There are a few brands in North America that are made with non-hydrogenated oil. These may be used sparingly, but do remember that they are still 100% fat.

Try the following as acceptable alternatives for your morning toast.

All-fruit spreads: "conserves," without the refined sugars of "preserves," jams, or jellies.

Apple butter or apple sauce: sprinkled with cinnamon.

Avocado: particularly good on bagels. High fat content.

Nut butters: High fat content. Good for growing children especially or those adults who need to gain weight.

Tahini: sesame seed paste. High fat content.

Extra virgin olive oil or flax seed oil: available in refrigerator case of natural food store, brushed lightly on toast. 100% fat, albeit "good" fat.

Coconut-Flax Butter*

I have provided you with many breakfast ideas but the list goes on... Use your imagination. Leftovers from the night before can be included in a fast, healthy breakfast. Many of us love leftover cold pizza in the morning or include leftover steamed vegetables with a tofu scramble. A non-fat fruit crisp or rice pudding that you had for dessert the night before can now serve as a delicious breakfast.

Can anyone still say, "I don't know what to have for breakfast"?

* Recipe in Recipe Collection

Chapter Three

~Lunches and Dinners

The strategy for preparing lunch and dinner is basically the same and the two meals are interchangeable. In fact a quick and easy lunch idea is to prepare leftovers from the previous night's dinner.

Planning a Well-Balanced Meal

A well-balanced lunch or dinner contains the following foods.

A starched-based entrée (grains, pasta, or potato/squash dish) with or without a concentrated protein complement like legumes, nuts, or seeds

Green and yellow vegetables as side dishes

An optional dessert such as fresh fruit

At least 50% of the food in these meals should be raw. A vegetable salad of some type would ideally help meet this goal. Fresh vegetables are vital for their vitamin, mineral and live enzyme content.

More Good Meal Ideas

Soups and stews are versatile, delicious entrées to prepare for lunch or dinner. They can be made with a wide variety of healthy ingredients, from grains and vegetables to legumes and seeds, and served with hearty whole-grain bread. Plus, soups travel well in a thermos and are ideal heated for the next day's lunch. Make a large potful for the refrigerator and enjoy it over several days.

You will also want to experiment with a wide variety of pasta and whole grain preparation techniques. Finally start experimenting with a wide variety of salads, from small side salads to large dinner salads with high-protein nuts and seeds and top with some great-tasting low-oil dressings (see recipes). Remember, the more colors in the salad the healthier it is.

Cooking with Baked Potatoes

Potatoes are a wonderful "power" food. They are dense, filling, full of nutrients and come in a variety of shapes, sizes, colors and tastes. I recommend you try all of them. Do try to buy them organic so that you do not have to peel them and can eat the very nutritious potato skin. You can steam potatoes, bake them and cook them in soups and stews. A simple steamed or baked potato can be transformed into a sumptuous entrée by adding toppings. Here are some ideas.

Potato Topping Ideas

Fresh salsa for Mexican-style potatoes
Extra virgin olive oil or flax seed oil drizzled on top
Non-dairy gravy*
Soy yogurt and chives
Salad greens with low-oil or oil-free salad dressing
Chili* or baked beans*
Steamed greens or broccoli florets with a dash of balsamic vinegar
Marinara Sauce* bottled or Vegetarian Spaghetti Sauce*
Sautéed mushrooms
Vegetable curry*
Ratatouille*

It is always a good idea to have plenty of leftover steamed or baked potatoes and yams on hand because they are fat-free and very versatile. Use them straight from the fridge as a snack or in the following dishes.

Slice and dice them and add to soups and casseroles.

Chop them along with onions and green peppers and sauté in non-stick pan with spices for delicious hash browns.

Cook and chill red and white new potatoes and add to salads.

Transform cooked potatoes into potato salad.

Tips for Easy Food Preparation

Set aside an evening or afternoon to prepare foods for freezing or storing. This will make meal preparation later in the week much easier and faster.

Prepare a big pot of vegetable stew to keep in the refrigerator and eat over several days. Keep adding fresh vegetables to the stew as well as the water in which you cook any vegetables in order to recapture the minerals lost to the cooking water.

Make a large whole-grain or pasta casserole and freeze in individual containers for later lunches and dinners.

Bake a dozen potatoes for snacks and meal supplements – filling and fat-free.

Use a rice cooker to prepare a large pot of rice, barley, millet or other favorite grain to keep in the refrigerator and add to stews, soups and sandwich spreads during the week.

* Recipe in Recipe Collection

Peel and slice a batch of fresh vegetables like carrots, daikon, broccoli and cucumbers and store in individual plastic bags to take with you for snacks. You can eat as much of these fat-free, high-fiber foods as you want during the day!

Lunch Ideas

Besides the usual lunches centered around the previous night's dinner entrée, try the following ideas for quick and nutritious mid-day meals.

Thick vegetable soup and whole grain bread
Large salads and soup
Raw vegetables and non-dairy dip
Baked potatoes and yams with sauces and salads
Corn on the cob: serve with soup or salad
Make grain salads by adding diced vegetables and oil-free salad dressings to favorite grains such as bulgur, barley, millet.

Sandwich Ideas

For tasty lunches that are not based on the previous night's dinner, explore the Sandwich section of the Recipe Collection. You will find that you can make sandwiches an "art form," with delicious ideas like chick-pea spread with tomatoes and sprouts in pocket pita bread, or tofu spread on whole wheat bread with lettuce, tomatoes and "all the trimmings." Over fourteen different sandwich wraps are described.

Lettuce and Nut Butter Sandwich: this combination may sound strange to the "uninitiated" but lettuce goes well with nut butter. The lettuce provides a nice crunch and the water content offsets the dryness of the nut butter. Cucumbers work well too as well as shredded carrots.

Sack Lunches

For those of you who prefer to take you lunch to work here are some great ideas for keeping your Transition foods crisp and tasty until you are ready to enjoy them.

Invest in an insulated "lunch box." Most department stores now carry wonderful "lunch boxes" made of nylon pack cloth with high-tech insulation. Many designs include heavy-duty two-way zippers, elastic straps to hold utensils and a pocket for a little "blue ice" pouch. Keep at your desk at work and munch away!

Invest in a wide-mouth thermos. Carry tasty hot soup, stew or chili with you. To retain more heat first fill the thermos with very hot water then empty and fill with food. Also, you might want to wrap the thermos in a towel for extra insulation.

Save your small plastic containers, like those from soy yogurt. These containers are ideal for packing fragile vegetables such as tomatoes. Bring along a sharp knife and slice these vegetables on your sandwich or into your salad just before you eat it.

Buy reusable plastic "zip-lock" bags. Lettuce leaves stay a lot crisper outside the sandwich. Take the lettuce in a separate plastic bag and add to your sandwich just before you eat it.

Tofu Ideas

Try the following ideas:

Cube and marinate tofu in soy sauce or favorite marinate then add it to vegetable stir-fries and sautés instead of meats, poultry or fish.

Mash it with tahini, tamari, tumeric and chopped onions as a scrambled egg substitute or to create a tofu spread.

Blend tofu into gravies.

Use it blended with water as a binder in cake batters.

Marinate, slice and sauté tofu.

Bread it as "cutlets."

Blend tofu with fruit and fruit juice for an instant "yogurt."

Use tofu to make "sour cream," "ricotta cheese," and "cream cheese."

Look up and try the delicious tofu recipes in this book.

Chapter Four

~Using Healthy Ingredients

Meat, Poultry and Fish Replacements

Instead of hamburgers, try soy, grain or Vegetable Burgers*

Instead of hot dogs, try tofu dogs.

Instead of meatloaf try NeatLoaf*, a savory mixture of cooked grains, nuts, lentils and vegetables.

In most bean soups, chilis and stews you do not need to replace the meat, just leave it out. If you want to replace it try:

Lentils

Frozen and thawed tofu (for a spongy, chewy texture)

Marinated and baked tofu (for a firm, chewy texture)

Seitan (meat-like ingredient made from wheat gluten and seasonings, see glossary)

Tempeh (cultured soy product, see glossary)

Replace beef, chicken or fish broth with vegetable broth, stock or water.

Replace ground meat in dishes like "Sloppy Joes," chili, or stuffed green peppers with cooked grains such as brown rice, bulgur wheat, or flavored soy-based granules, called Texturized Vegetable Protein, or "TVP".

Replace meats and fish in stir-fries with nuts, or chewy vegetables like shiitake mushrooms, eggplant cubes, green beans, and potatoes.

Dairy Replacements in Recipes

Instead of milk use:

Soy milk: (plain) in the same proportions

Rice Dream: rice milk (somewhat sweeter) dilute 1 part water to 3 to 4 parts Rice Dream

Nut milks: cashew cream instead of whipping cream

Apple juice: in sweet recipes like cakes and muffins

Sunny Milk*

Banana milk*

* Recipe in Recipe Collection

Instead of margarine and butter use:

Unrefined, heat-resistant, expeller-pressed oils such as extra virgin olive or almond for cooking and baking.

Extra virgin olive oil, pistachio oil, Coconut-Flax Butter* or flaxseed oil: try brushing any of these on your corn on the cob.

Try flaxseed, sunflower or walnut oil lightly brushed over raw or steamed vegetables or grains

Coconut-Flax Butter*: as a spread or for baking

Non-hydrogenated margarine

Instead of sour cream or yogurt use:

Soy-based sour cream or soy yogurt, home-made or from natural food store.

Instead of cheese use:

Soy cheese: cholesterol-free, but still contains fat and casein, a milk protein that can cause dairy-related problems. A "novelty" transition food.

Very firm tofu or crumbled and seasoned is a particularly good replacement for ricotta cheese in recipes such as lasagna.

Instead of Eggs

Eggs provide different properties in different recipes so successful conversions depend on the type of recipe you are using.

Typically ¼ cup firm tofu (blended with small amount of water) replaces 1 egg. This conversion works well for quiches, omelets, scrambled eggs and pie fillings.

In baked goods, such as muffins, quick breads and cakes, replace 1 egg with any of the following:

¼ cup soft tofu blended until smooth in a blender with other liquid ingredients

1 T flax seeds with ¼ cup water blended at high speed for 1 to 2 minutes in a blender until thick and frothy like beaten eggs, fold into the batter gently

Ener-G powdered egg replacer (found in natural food stores)

A banana blended with ¼ cup water

Soft Drink Replacements

Fresh fruit and vegetable juices are healthy and delicious and can easily be made with a good juicer. If you do not have time to wash and juice your

*Recipe in Recipe Collection

own fresh produce, try good quality, dated, fresh juices found in the refrigerator cases of most natural food stores.

Mineral water alone, or with a squeeze of lemon, lime or orange.

For a sweeter taste, mix mineral water half and half with your favorite organic fruit juice. As your diet and tastes change you may find that bottled fruit juices are too sweet for you. Diluted half and half with either mineral (sparkling) water or plain water they make a nice beverage with only half the calories and simple sugars.

Other Substitutions

Instead of 1 cup all-purpose white flour try:

$^3/_4$ cup coarse whole wheat flour

or

$^3/_4$ cup barley flour

or

$^7/_8$ cup whole wheat pastry flour

or

$^3/_4$ cup buckwheat flour

Instead of sautéing in oil:

Sauté using water, water and natural soy sauce or vegetable stock

Bake using applesauce or water instead of oil

Instead of sugar use the following for pie crusts/cookies:

Brown rice syrup, barley malt syrup, maple syrup or applesauce

Date sugar, dates or raisins

Grains

How many grains can you name? Most people can name two to four, but there are so many more and I encourage you to try them all: oats, millet, quinoa, amaranth, corn, rye, spelt, wheat, triticale, buckwheat, barley, kamut, couscous, kasha and rice – not just rice, but long grain brown rice, short grain brown rice, sweet brown rice, basmati brown rice and so forth. So many choices!

Since you will be using grains as an important part of many of your dinner and luncheon menus you will want to vary them as much as possible.

Basic Recipe for Cooking Grains

Rinse all whole grains before cooking to remove tiny stones or other field substances. Measure the grain before you wash it.

The most common way to cook grain is to steep it. This entails bringing the water to a boil, adding the grain, covering and simmering for anywhere from 15 minutes to an hour and a half depending on the type of grain.

1. Use approximately 2 cups water to 1 cup grain except for millet use a 3 to 1 ratio.

2. In a quart pot bring water to boil, add grain, cover and simmer on a low heat until water is absorbed.

3. When grain is done remove from heat, uncover pot and allow to cool without stirring.

GRAIN(1 CUP)	WATER (CUPS)	TIME(MIN.)	INSTRUCTIONS
Amaranth	2½ – 3	10-25	
Barley	3	50-55	
Buckwheat Groats	2	15-20	toast first
Millet	2½	35-40	toast first
Oats (Rolled)	¾-1½	5-10	water and time depend on desired texture
Brown Rice	2¼	40	
Wheat Berries	3½ – 4	55-60	soak 12 hours

Ideas for Adding Variety to Your Grain Dishes

Add some nuts (walnuts, pecans, almonds) to the cooking water and cook the grain with the nuts. Add a few more nuts just before serving.

Add some seeds (sunflower, sesame, caraway, pumpkin) to the cooking water. If you want roast the seeds lightly in the oven before adding

Cook the grain with chopped vegetables like onions, corn, celery, chunked squash or root vegetables like carrots or parsnips.

Add some herbs and spices to the cooking water. Try tamari, vegetable bouillon or classic spices like sage, basil and oregano. Experiment!

Cook combinations of grains. Mix rice with barley, millet, rye or bulgur.

Cook the grains with legumes. Use beans or chickpeas (garbanzo beans) from jar or can. Add lentils to the grain just before cooking. Grains can be roasted lightly in the oven before cooking for a firmer texture and a nut-like flavor.

Cook the grains with leftovers and freshen with chopped celery, walnuts, onions and tamari. Cook in a covered pan.

Cook with sea vegetables to increase trace mineral content. Try dulse, arame, kombu. (See glossary under Sea Vegetables.) All are available at natural food stores.

You can also vary your grain dishes by serving them with a gravy or sauce. For example:

Use a starch-based ingredient for the gravy such as a little arrowroot, kuzu (see glossary), or oat flour browned in a pan. Mix with water, tamari and spices.

Serve with tomato-based sauces and miso-based stocks.

Use gravies based on nutritional yeast or tahini.

Almost all the ideas for potato toppings can be used successfully with the grain of your choice.

Cooking with Brown Rice

Cook up a big pot of rice and use it in a variety of ways throughout the week. To heat and refresh it use a steamer.

Experiment with brown rice. Try using it in soups, casseroles, pilafs, stir-fries, grain salads and desserts like puddings and pies.

Try making a pie crust by pressing cooked rice into a pie shell and baking for fifteen minutes. Then fill it with vegetable mixture or wheat meat (seitan) for a delicious pie.

Using Beans and Other Legumes

Now that you know more about grains let us look at another very important food family that you will be using on your Transition Plan: legumes. As we mentioned earlier, a legume is anything that grows in a pod. Legumes are a primary source of protein in the Transition Plan diet and are of best use to the body when eaten with whole grains (2½ parts grain to 1 part legume).

The legume clan is a large one. Take advantage of its variety: navy beans, aduki beans, pinto beans, chickpeas (garbanzo beans), green peas, many varieties of lentils, and alfalfa sprouts, to name a few.

Try using legumes in the following ways:

Add to soups, stews and salads.

Soak, rinse, cook and mash them. Then season with garlic and spices for high protein spreads to replace meats on your sandwiches – great for growing children!

Substitute them for dairy-based dips. Just soak, rinse, cook and mash (or purée with liquid for desired consistency) and season to taste. For example: bean dip and beans spreads.

For Individuals Concerned with Intestinal Gas

Soak your legumes overnight. Then discard the soaking water and rinse thoroughly before you make your bean soup or chili. You will wash away much of the bean sugars that can contribute to intestinal gas. You can also use a few drops of an enzyme product called Beano available at most natural food stores and said to be very effective. Most intestinal gas is swallowed air. Chewing each mouthful "to a cream" will force out excess air and most "gas problems" will disappear.

Green Leafy Vegetables

Green leafy vegetables are nutritional champions, rich in calcium, iron, beta carotene, low in sodium and calories – and the darker the green the more nutritious. Try to include them in at least two meals per day. They are easy to cook (steam them for 3 to 5 minutes and serve with lemon juice or sauce) but most can be eaten raw, and some are available frozen.

To add variety to your meals, you will want to expand your repertoire of green leafy vegetables beyond iceberg lettuce (the least nutritious) to broccoli, kale, collards, Swiss chard, mustard and beet greens, and occasionally spinach. Once you have found your local farmer's market take some time to familiarize yourself with the wide variety of produce available.

Cooking Greens

Follow these suggestions when cooking with greens.

Do not throw away the outer leaves as these are usually the greenest and most nutritious.

To obtain maximum nutritional benefit most should be eaten raw or lightly steamed.

Older, strongly-flavored greens like collards and mustard or turnip greens can benefit from longer cooking in a seasoned broth. To lessen the bitter taste, plunge them into a pot of boiling water for 2-4 minutes.

Varying the greens in your salads, casseroles and rice dishes will add taste variety as well as texture.

Tips for Getting the Fat Out of Your Cooking

Instead of oil-based salad dressing, use a sweet rice vinegar.

Instead of cream sauces, use tomato salsa for topping on potatoes and other veggies.

Instead of vegetable fats, sauté foods in water or vegetable broth.

Instead of butter or margarine, use fruit spreads on toast.

Try baking, steaming, sautéing or stir-frying using water or vegetable broth. Avoid deep-fat frying all together.

Cooking with Oils

While you are advised to keep your oil consumption to a minimum (less than a tablespoon a day) you may still want to occasionally cook with it. Follow these simple steps.

Use the smallest amount of oil possible for each dish.

Cook at low temperatures.

Never let the oil smoke in a skillet. When you see oil smoking it means the oil is breaking down into harmful, cell-damaging free radicals.

When stir-frying, heat the skillet up to cooking temperature then add oil and *immediately* add vegetables. Remember: "hot wok, cold oil."

Mixing the oil 1 to 1 with water before heating will keep the temperature down in the skillet.

The oils that are best for cooking (most heat-tolerant) are coconut, almond, peanut and sesame, in that order.

Herbs, Spices And Seasonings

A wide variety of herbs, spices, and seasonings are your most important ingredients for enhancing your whole food diet as you phase out the fats, salt and sugar in your foods. They also provide you with the opportunity to be creative in the kitchen so experiment and have fun!

To add a salty flavor try:

Celery: fresh, seed or powder
Garlic: fresh, granulated or powder
Hot spices: cayenne, chili or Tabasco
Lemon: juice or peel
Onion: fresh, flakes or powder
Parsley: fresh or dried

To add a sweet flavor, try:

Allspice	Mace
Cardamom	Mint
Cinnamon	Nutmeg
Cloves	Vanilla extract
Ginger	

Seasonings Used in Ethnic Dishes

French:

tarragon, nutmeg

Italian:

oregano, basil, fennel, rosemary, garlic, parsley, marjoram

Mexican:

chili powder, chili pepper flakes, cumin, cilantro, oregano

Chinese:

ginger, star anise, fennel, curry, cayenne, cilantro, hot mustard, garlic

German and Scandinavian:

caraway, dill, cinnamon, cardamom, paprika, garlic, lemon

Indian:

cumin, curry, coriander, turmeric, fenugreek, garlic, saffron, cinnamon

Chapter Five

~ Smart Shopping

Before you step foot in the supermarket, you have to know what items you are planning to buy. So, let us consider the following.

Meal Planning Tips

Whether you are cooking for yourself or a family, every cook knows that it can sometimes be a difficult task to prepare a meal "from scratch" especially for today's busy homemakers. Try these tips to make your meal planning and cooking time as productive as possible.

Take time to plan your meals and prepare your shopping list at the beginning of each week.

Keep meal plans simple especially if you are pressed for time. For example, if you cook up grains or potatoes, add steamed vegetables, fresh vegetables or a sauce, and you have a complete meal.

For variety and enjoyment, make use of sauces. Change the sauce and you have changed the meal.

Start your meal with fresh vegetables either raw in a salad or as fresh juice.

Cook foods such as beans, soups, lasagnas and casseroles ahead of time and freeze in serving portions.

Use spices and herbs according to your taste when trying recipes.

Vary your grains, beans and vegetables. Variety is the spice of life and the key to enjoyment and better health.

Vary your meals with the seasons. Consider more warming foods in winter like soups and stews, and more cooling foods in summer like fruit bowls and smoothies.

Have a breakfast or lunch for dinner.

Use a crockpot to cook soups or stews during the day while you are at work.

Smart Shopping Rules

Never go shopping when you are hungry. Hunger makes you want to buy everything in sight, something your wallet, your waistline and your arteries can not afford.

31

Since the shelflife of most store-bought produce is 3 to 4 days, plan to shop about two times a week. (Note: locally grown produce at the farmer's market usually lasts longer.)

Resist popular processed foods that are overloaded with refined sweeteners, saturated fats, preservatives and additives. These foods occupy most of the center of the supermarket shelves; most of the health-supporting whole foods tend to be on the periphery of the stores. The less time spent roaming these lifeless center aisles, the better.

Always try to buy organic to get more nutrient value and fewer pesticides from your produce.

Label Reading Made Easy

Any "smart shopper" is an avid label reader. This is an essential habit to form because many of the processed or prepared foods that we buy contain too much fat, refined sugars and hidden animal products.

Fortunately, because you are going to be buying predominantly fresh whole foods, very little label reading will be needed but some will still be necessary and you need to know what to look for. The more common packaged goods you will likely be buying (and thus labels you will be reading) are jars of spaghetti sauce, or beans or chickpeas (garbanzo beans) ready to add to a salad. You should also check the label of any frozen dinner or packaged spread or dairy substitute as well as every loaf of whole grain bread or other baked goods.

Reading labels in the Transition Plan style is easy. You are mostly looking to see that the ingredients are natural and wholesome. In general the fewer words on a package label the better. A label on a peanut butter jar should read "Fresh whole peanuts" and that is all. Stay away from foods with labels that include, sucrose, molasses, high fructose corn syrup, (all aliases for sugar), partially hydrogenated vegetable oils, or any words that you can not pronounce or you do not understand.

You are definitely checking the label for:

1. Cholesterol per serving: Dealing with cholesterol levels is simple since all plant-based foods are cholesterol-free, the cholesterol amount per serving should ideally read "0." Cholesterol you do not eat is cholesterol your liver doesn't have to excrete, and thus, that much less to clog your arteries. The maximum cholesterol our body can excrete is between only 100 milligrams to 300 milligrams each day – and that should be cholesterol your own body makes, so the less eaten the better, and none is best.

2. Fat per serving: Excessive fats are to be avoided. Read the labels for the grams of fat in each serving. Beware if a single serving has more than 5 grams of fat. Each gram of fat equals 9 calories. Limit your total fat intake to 20% of your total calories and no more than 10% if you are trying to lose weight or have any degenerative condition.

3. Hidden animal products: Check labels for hidden ingredients of animal origin: common aliases for milk products are casein, sodium caseinate, whey, skim milk powder, buttermilk powder and all can cause allergic reactions in those sensitive to milk protein; tallow and lard; offending animal protein can be found in beef extract and gelatin.

4. Preservatives, additives, hydrogenated oils and other chemicals: Be on the lookout. If there are two or more words on the label that are not the names of fruits, vegetables or other natural ingredients you know, reconsider if you really want it in your body. No one knows the effects these chemicals have in our cells and you shouldn't have to be part of an experiment to find out. Look for the same food in a more natural, wholefood form.

Remember that many of the most nutritious foods have no labels at all, for example, fresh whole foods like fruits, vegetables, bulk grains, beans and potatoes. Try to purchase locally-grown organic produce as much as possible. There is no substitute for fresh, natural, whole food.

Health-Focused Shopping List

Power Foods:

> Grains, cereals, breads
> Pastas
> Legumes

Vital Foods:

> Vegetables
> Fruits

Helpful Additions:

> Oils
> Flour, thickeners, leavening agents
> Sweeteners
> Dried fruits, nuts
> Seasonings, herbs and spices
> Sea vegetables
> Condiments, sauces
> Miscellaneous

A Blueprint for Successful Shopping

1. Enter the store with your **Health Focused Shopping List** in hand, and:

2. Find and select the Power Foods you need, like whole grains and pastas, breads and cereals.

3. Then complement the Power Foods by picking concentrated protein foods like jars of beans and lentils, as well as almond and other nut butters. Do not forget tasty sauces, flavorings and useful oils, like extra virgin olive and other unrefined oils.

4. Pick up the living Vital Foods in the produce section of the market: green and yellow vegetables and fruits and potatoes.

5. Fill any ingredient gaps in recipes or meal planning with filler items like canned, prepared or frozen foods from non-dairy spreads to soy milk and frozen tofu lasagna dinners.

6. *Then leave the store* before you yield to unhealthful temptations!

Your Local Natural Foods Store

Anyone embarking on the Transition Plan must pay a visit to a nearby natural food store. A nutritional treasure chest awaits you there as you see all the alternative products available for sandwich fillings and dinner entrées, from soy based "hot dogs" and grain-based "burgers" to frozen Italian-style meat-free entrées.

The produce department usually offers a wonderful array of locally-grown, unsprayed, organic Vital Foods, as well as economic bulk buys on whole grains, pastas, cereals and other staple foods like tahini, tamari and nutritional yeast. Have sealed jars or other containers at home to store these bulk foods.

The refrigerator case will have fresh tofu, soy based yogurts and the meat-like soy and grain-derived products for sandwiches. You will also want to explore the available dairy substitutes. There are now non-dairy products on the market to replace everything from milk and ice cream to sour cream and mayonnaise. The freezer case will have frozen vegetarian dinner entrées and taste-tempting, non-dairy desserts.

The staff at most natural food stores are usually delighted to guide you to the products you need. However, it is a good idea to take an experienced friend with you on your first shopping excursion if you can.

The Local Farmer's Market

Also try to find a farmer's market near you where you can buy high-quality Vital Foods at bargain prices, as well as meet other health-minded, bargain-seeking people like yourself.

Buying and Storing Oils

While you are not going to have a lot of oils in your refrigerator they are worth mentioning because there are arguments for and against the use of small amounts of unrefined oils like extra virgin olive or almond oils. While they add flavor and taste satisfaction to the diet, excessive amounts may add to weight problems, impede blood circulation and possibly increase risk for some cancers. Limit intake of oils to no more than two tablespoons a day.

In the Plan, the fats needed for normal body function, such as skin oils and hormone synthesis, are almost exclusively derived from wholefood sources like whole grains, seeds, nuts and olives.

If you decide to use extracted oils in your diet, remember that all oils go rancid in the presence of light, heat, and air. Therefore:

Buy only unrefined oils packed in dark bottles or cans. Avoid "all purpose vegetable oil" in clear plastic bottles as they have been exposed to light for long periods of time in the store.

Keep opened oils in a cool, dark place. You may store your oils in the refrigerator, but olive oil will need time to liquefy at room temperature before using.

Buy oils in small containers and use them rapidly. A gallon can of olive oil is no bargain if it takes you ten months to use it and the last quart is rancid!

Always purchase the highest quality oils that are marked "unrefined." This means that no chemicals and very little heat was used in the extraction process.

Equipping Your Kitchen

Let us talk a little about how to equip your kitchen. Just as a master craftsperson knows that the right tools are essential for building a beautiful house, so, too, the right utensils, tools and ingredients are necessary for proper nutrition, not only to create healthy meals, but also to be efficient, and to keep food preparation fun.

The following list identifies the type of utensils and appliances that you are likely to use to prepare your Transition Plan meals. You probably already own many of these items. However, if you must purchase any of them, consider it an investment in your health and your future.

Kitchen Utensils and Appliances

"Essential" Items:

Blender

Chopping boards: one for vegetables and one for fruit

A good set of kitchen knives

Stainless steel vegetable steamer (a simple basket model will do)

Non-stick pots and skillets: stainless steel, glass or cast iron

Baking pans and sheets(stainless steel, glass, or non-stick): for cakes, casseroles, pies, cookies and muffins

Extras: While these appliances are not essential they make food preparation much easier and will liberate you from unnecessary hours in the kitchen.

Wok: with a long handle for comfort

Toaster Oven

Food processor: for "instant" salads, spreads and such

Juice extractor: for fresh vitamin/mineral packed juices

Crockpot (slow cooker): for cooking soups and stews while you are out

Electric rice cooker: for perfect, hassle-free rice and other grains

Pressure cooker: to shorten cooking time for such things as beans, potatoes and stews

Waffle iron

Food Dehydrator

Chapter Six

~Dining Out

You may be saying to yourself that it is easy to eat in this style in the privacy of your own home, but you will never be able to do it when you go out to eat. If you feel that way you will be happy to know that "eating out" and "eating healthy" are no longer mutually exclusive. In fact, ordering a healthy, cholesterol-free meal in any restaurant is becoming easier all the time. With an increasingly diverse mixture of ethnic restaurants to choose from there is no reason why you cannot continue your Transition Plan every time you go out to eat.

Creative Ordering

The only difference for Transition Plan restaurant ordering is that you need to study the menu a little more carefully. You are still going to be eating Power Foods and Vital Foods; you just need to think more creatively about how to order and coordinate your meal.

Be sure to look at all categories on the menu not just entrées. The appetizers, salads, soups and side dishes sections, may each offer cholesterol-free dishes that you can combine for your entrée.

Most dishes can be easily and deliciously prepared free of animal products if you but request it. Ask and you shall receive!

A Common Mistake

A common mistake that most people make when they go out to dinner is to "save their appetite" for the restaurant. The problem with this approach is that most people are so hungry when they get to the restaurant that they begin to gorge themselves on white-flour dinner rolls and butter.

Alternatively, plan your eating day wisely. Even though you are going to a restaurant for dinner, have something to eat before you go out to the restaurant: a piece of fruit or some whole grain bread, anything nutritious and a little filling so that you do not arrive at the restaurant famished.

Restaurant Ordering Guidelines

Here are some suggestions for ordering in different types of restaurants.

Italian

Salad usually on the menu under "Insalata."

Dark green lettuce can be mixed with tomatoes, garlic, basil, olives and mushrooms. Ask for a non-dairy Italian dressing on the side.

Zuppa rustica: a tangy tomato vegetable soup.

Antipasto appetizers: includes small cheeseless pizza, called "focaccia," made with tomatoes, garlic, basil and olives.

Pastas with tomato and mushroom sauce: (may be called marinara sauce) can also be ordered "primavera style" with fresh garden vegetables in the sauce or other ingredients such as dried tomatoes, onions, leeks, garlic and greens.

Side dishes: can include "melanzani" a sautéed eggplant with onions and basil, topped with marinara sauce and "gnocci," seasoned potato-filled dumplings.

Pizza! Just ask them to hold the cheese and add extra tomato sauce and ingredients like sun-dried tomatoes, mushrooms onions, bell peppers, fresh basil, garlic, olives and other vegetables like broccoli and artichoke hearts. You will be surprised how delicious this is!

Chinese

Steamed rice and traditional Chinese tea go well with all the following meals. Let the waiter know that you do not want any of your dishes made with eggs, chicken broth or monosodium glutamate (MSG).

Salads made with lettuce, onion, tomato and cucumber with a rice vinegar dressing. You can follow this with a clear, non-meat-based vegetable soup.

Vegetable chow meins served over steamed rice or noodles.

Boost the protein value of a dish by requesting Power Foods from the nut or legume family like cashews, almonds, tofu or snow peas.

Tofu dishes may be listed as "bean curd." Look for them and enjoy them.

In addition to being served cubed and added to stir-fried vegetables, tofu may be marinated and turned into mock meat dishes with the texture and taste closely resembling chicken, pork or beef.

Sautéed broccoli and snow peas with cashews

Asparagus with tofu and black mushroom

Mixed vegetables in garlic sauce

Vegetable fried rice

Spicy Szechwan-style noodles

A delightful light sweet dessert – lychee nuts in light syrup

Japanese

Ask the waiter to be sure that no meat, fish or eggs are used, even in the broths.

Cucumber salad

A broth soup like miso or sunomono

Rice and vegetables in several forms:

> Vegetable sukiyaki

> Vegetarian sushi – cucumber rolls, california rolls without crab

Soba noodles made from buckwheat

Mexican

Beware that the tortilla chips may contain hydrogenated oils and the beans may be cooked in lard. That is why it is a good idea to check with the restaurant ahead of time and ask if your food can be cooked without any fat. Be sure to ask them to hold the cheese.

Vegetable salad

Gazpacho: a cold tomato and vegetable soup

Use beans and/or rice instead of meat for filler (hold the cheese) with the following:

> Corn tortillas

> Enchiladas

> Burritos

> Tacos

Side orders of Mexican rice mixed with black beans

Avocado-based guacamole

Salsa on tacos and vegetables

East Indian

Meals are typically served with flat whole wheat bread called "chappatis." Avoid butter on the chappatis as well as other breads like "poori," which are deep fried.

Appetizers like vegetable samosa, a thin layered pastry stuffed with mixed vegetables

Mulligatawny soup: flavorful vegetables in a rich stock

Dal: lentil stews, which can be seasoned from mild to spicy

Rice-based dishes: served with colorful vegetables and savory flavorings like sweet mango chutney

Vegetable curries: including spinach and potatoes, pea and cauliflower, and others served in curry sauces

"Masala dosa": crepes prepared from rice and lentils, stuffed with vegetables

Chickpeas cooked with fresh herbs
Long grain Basmati rice served with mixed vegetables

Thai

"Pad Thai" noodles with vegetable. You may need to remind the waiter to leave out the chicken and any egg
Tangy lemon/ginger soup: usually made with chicken but if you request it can be made deliciously with tofu
Spinach with black bean sauce
Baby corn sautéed with mushrooms
Mixed vegetable curry or broccoli sautéed with bean sprouts

Greek, Israeli or Middle Eastern

Greek-style salads with many varieties of lettuce, tomatoes, onion, garlic and Greek olives. Just ask the waiter to leave out the "feta" goat milk cheese. Many of the rice-based dishes normally served with lamb or chicken can be made with vegetables instead.
"Baba ghanooj": a dip made of eggplant, sesame butter, lemon juice and a bit of garlic, garnished with onions and tomatoes
Chick pea spread called "hummus" with flat, round, whole wheat pita bread
"Tabouli": a cold bulgur wheat salad seasoned with herbs and mint
Side dishes: try grape leaves or cabbage rolls stuffed with seasoned rice.

Vegetarian and Natural Foods

Dinner salads: carrot, spinach, mixed green
Non-meat burger sandwiches
Black bean chili
Spinach lasagna
Vegetable soups, such as thick split pea served with dark bread
Shepherds pie with mashed potatoes and vegetable stew
Fresh fruit and vegetable juices: carrot-beet-celery, fruit smoothies such as frozen banana, pineapple, mango and papaya

Fast Foods

Salad bars, but steer clear of dairy/high fat dressings. Look for low-cal Italian dressing or fresh lemons to squeeze over your salad.
Baked potatoes with salsa.
Burger sandwich with lettuce, tomato, mustard, ketchup etc., but ask them to hold the meat!

American/Continental

Although the following suggestions may seem an awkward way to order a meal, be patient. These are times of transition for our whole society. More and more restaurants are adding entire meatless entrée sections to their menu and cholesterol-free dining is becoming easier. The more we ask for these kinds of dishes, the more there will be.

Check the appetizer section of the menu for the following:

Vegetable platter with non-dairy dip

Stuffed sautéed mushrooms

Marinated asparagus spears

Garden or warm spinach salad: avoid warm dressings containing bacon and remind them to leave out any condiments such as shrimp, cheese or bacon.

Side dishes of carrots, olives or broccoli florets with non-dairy dressing like Italian or oil and vinegar. For a change of pace ask for salsa or guacamole dip instead.

Baked potatoes stuffed with broccoli and salsa. Have several for your main course!

Bean soups made with vegetable stock

Pasta and rice dishes

A vegetable soup with whole-grain bread, salad and side dishes of lightly steamed green and yellow vegetables can be the basis for a filling and satisfying meal.

For Breakfast choose:

Fruit, orange juice, half a grapefruit, or fruit salad

Cereals: including oatmeal, granolas, mueslix-style cereals and commercial flake cereals, topped with fruit

Oatmeal with raisins and cinnamon

To pour over your cereal, try fruit juice like apple, pineapple or even orange. Some people bring a small container of flavored soy milk with them to put on their cereal.

Hash brown potatoes (baked, not fried with oil) with ketchup and whole wheat toast with fruit preserves or jams

Tips for the Traveler

Traveling can sometimes present unique challenges to the nutritious eater. However more and more carriers are offering vegetable platters, especially airlines. Check with your travel agent when you are booking reservations and ask for non-dairy, vegetarian style meals.

In addition you might want to bring your own little satchel of wholesome foods such as rice cakes, fruits, trail mixes and popcorn. These items are instant, convenient and they travel well.

For lunches on the road bring pita bread stuffed with fresh vegetables and nut butters or tahini.

When traveling by car, bus or train, you may also want to bring screw top containers with:

Boxes of instant hummus and instant black bean dip (Fantastic Foods or other brands) – just add water.

Fresh drinking water

Tamari, Bragg Liquid Aminos or another natural soy sauce

Utensils

So whether you are at home, on the road or in your favorite restaurant, a health supporting diet is available to you if you want it.

Chapter Seven

~Holidays, Snacks and Parties

Ideas for Entertaining

Focus on the real meaning of a holiday instead of getting caught up in serving rich and fattening foods.

When going to a dinner party, inform the host/hostess in advance that you are on a low-fat diet.

If you are sure that the foods at a party will all be fatty, plan to eat a mini-meal beforehand.

When invited to a potluck, offer to bring a cholesterol-free main dish. That way you can be confident there will be some food there that you can eat.

Volunteer to entertain more in my your home where you have control over the kitchen.

Purchase some vegetarian cookbooks that show how to make gourmet dishes.

The Real Meaning of Holidays

Before the feasting begins take a moment to reflect on the significance of the particular celebration. Whether it is a Thanksgiving celebration of the bountiful harvest, the spring Easter celebration of the renewal of life, the Passover recognition of the liberation of bondage or the Christmas rejoicing over the Personification of Love, remember that the focus is the joy in the heart, not the gorging of the stomach. Then, remember:

Fully enjoy the experience of being with family and friends.

Do not get into an argument over who is eating what.

Lovingly share your food and the decisions and choices you have made about your Transition Plan only if you are asked.

Do not judge anyone else or their food choices.

Be a glowing example of good health and let your appearance speak for you.

Holidays and parties are to enjoy, so enjoy!

Tips for Party Planning

If you have decided to plan a dinner party try the following ideas:

Consider hiring a natural foods caterer.

Pick up some or all of your dishes from a natural food store deli or from your favorite ethnic restaurant's take-out menu.

If you are a confident cook consult one of the gourmet vegetarian cookbooks and experiment with a new dish.

The Fourth of July or Canada Day Picnic

Sometimes casual events like a picnic can also be intimidating. The next time you are hosting that Fourth of July picnic, try serving:

Potato or macaroni salad, or coleslaw made with eggless mayonnaise

Tofu hot dogs

Tasty meatless burgers

Non-dairy ice cream treats and frozen fruit bars

Sparkling drinks with your favorite fruit juices and fizzy seltzer water

Super Bowl or Grey Cup Parties

And what about TV parties? Offer:

Baked tortilla chips with salsa or guacamole

Air-popped popcorn tossed with a little oil and seasoned salt

Vegetarian submarine sandwiches made with slices of seitan or thin-sliced tofu

Raw veggies like carrots and broccoli with non-dairy dips from your natural food store; make your own tofu, spinach, and toasted onion dip.

Mini pizzas topped with olives, mushrooms, onions, tomatoes and even pineapple, but hold the cheese!

Everyday Desserts

Everyday desserts from healthful fruit bowls to sinful tofu chocolate cheesecake, chocolate chip cookies and even moist devil's food cake can all be made without eggs, dairy products or other harmful ingredients. As long as they are enjoyed sparingly such taste treats certainly do not have to be banished from your life forever. Try some of the dessert recipes in this book.

Replacement for Dairy Treats

Natural food stores carry soy-based yogurts and ice cream substitutes such as Rice Dream.

Try the Tofu Yogurt* next time you get the desire for yogurt or an ice-cream-like treat.

Smoothies

What is as cool and delicious as a milkshake but with very little fat and no cholesterol? It is called a "banana smoothie" and its secret ingredient is frozen bananas. Next time you buy a bunch of bananas, peel several ripe ones and put them in an airtight container or plastic bag in the freezer. Be sure to use the frozen bananas within a month or two while they retain their light color.

When you are ready for a "milkshake" combine the following.

> One cup of liquid (try apple or other fruit juice, almond or soy milk or just plain water)
>
> 1 or 2 frozen bananas
>
> ½ t tahini
>
> a handful of fruit chunks of your choice (fresh or frozen berries, pear, fresh melon, papaya, dates).

Blend it all in a blender, adding extra water or ice chips if needed. A teaspoon of vanilla extract or a tablespoon of pure maple syrup may be added for extra sweetening, but is not necessary.

When you get the urge for ice cream, here are some cholesterol-free versions that can certainly "hit the spot".

Rice Dream frozen desserts by Imagine Foods are based on rice milk rather than cow's milk or cream. Available in natural food stores they come in pints or quarts and many flavors. This company also makes wonderful non-dairy ice cream treats.

Dates and Other Dried Fruits

These are great snack foods to keep handy in the refrigerator. Dates are naturally sweet and satisfy that occasional craving without excess fat and even with some measurable nutritional value.

Other dried fruits such as raisins, apricots, pears, peaches, and even cherries, papayas and mangoes, make tasty and healthy snacks. Choose the unsulfured varieties available in natural food stores whenever possible. It is a good idea to soak the dried fruits in order to re-hydrate them. Even though they may not look as good they will taste delicious and they are better for you without the preservative. Remember, however, that dried fruits are concentrated sweets so you will not want to eat too many at once, and remember to brush your teeth afterwards.

* Recipe in Recipe Collection

Snacks And In-a-Hurry Foods

It is only human nature to want to occasionally enjoy a mid-day, between-meal snack. Sometimes we are too busy to eat a full meal so we want something quick and nutritious to munch on. Next time you are in one of these moods try some of the following ideas.

Air-popped Popcorn: An air popper is well worth the modest investment. It is easy to use, needs no cleaning and pops reliably without burning the kernels. No oil is required so you avoid excess fat as well as the dangers associated with fats at high temperatures. After popping sprinkle popcorn with nutritional yeast, "Spike" or other powdered flavorings if desired.

Baked (not fried) tortilla chips and oil-free salsa: These tortilla chips are readily available in your natural food store. (Try a brand like Guiltless Gourmet.)

No-cholesterol nachos: These are a quick and satisfying meal in themselves as well as a great appetizer for guests. Place baked tortilla chips in overlapping layers to cover a baking pan. Mix up some Fantastic Foods instant refried beans or black beans (or use a can of vegetarian refried beans) and spoon on to the tortilla chips. Drizzle the oil-free salsa of your choice on top. If you want you can add additional condiments like jalapeno peppers, Greek peppers, roasted red peppers, chopped green chilis or black olives. Bake at 350ºF – 400ºF for 10-15 minutes until bubbly. If you do not mind the extra fat, you can top with a few dollops of guacamole before serving.

For more ideas for check the recipe section.

Chapter Eight

~Healthy Children

My son, Adam, chose to become a vegetarian when he was fourteen years old. A popular, athletic child, he found that this way of eating helped him to easily lose unwanted pounds and maintain his weight without dieting. It also helped to clear up his skin and make him a lot more attractive. For a teenager this spoke volumes.

I consider nourishing your children by providing and encouraging them to eat a healthy diet one of the greatest gifts of love that a parent can give. One of my saddest experiences is to find myself behind a parent with a child at a supermarket and see all the processed, high-fat, low-fiber, sugary foods that are in their shopping cart.

It should come as no surprise that the young, as well as the elderly, have special dietary needs that should be factored in when developing Transition Plan menus.

 I highly recommend "Pregnancy and Healthy Children" from *A Diet for All Reasons* audio Wellness Series, as well as Dr. Michael Klaper's book *Pregnancy, Children and the Vegan Diet*.

Special Dietary Considerations for Children

Children have special nutritional needs particularly in the early years. During the first one to two years breast milk is the perfect food with solid foods added beginning at about six months. Throughout their growing years they need a steady source of available protein, fat, iron, calcium and vitamins, especially B-12 and riboflavin.

During their first two years, children need proportionately more fat in their diet; a diet where nutritional fats make up 40% of the child's calorie intake is appropriate until age two. So do not begrudge them nut butters, avocados, bean spreads, etc. Taper the fat percentage down to 30% through their adolescent years, and down to 20% during the 'teens.

The smaller stomachs of children are easily filled with high-fiber foods. So, after weaning to table foods and throughout adolescence be sure your children's diets contain energy and protein-rich foods like crackers with nut spreads and whole grain pastas.

Contrary to popular belief it is a wise policy for children to avoid dairy products. This will protect them against allergies, asthma, eczema and anemia from intestinal bleeding, all known to be associated with dairy products in the diet.

Children's Parties

Children are sensitive to peer pressure so it is only natural they want to be part of the crowd. And there's no reason they cannot be when you serve the following dishes at your child's next party.

Pizzas or pastas made without meat and cheese (with extra sauce!)

Non-meat hot dogs and burgers served with ketchup, mustard, relish and all the trimmings.

Cakes made without eggs or dairy products

Non-dairy "ice cream" from the natural food store

Bowls of nut and raisin mix

Dried fruit and non-fat cookies from the natural food store

Feeding Young People

The best way to teach is by example. Provide the best foods you can, and enjoy them with your family. Experiment with different recipes and include your children.

Remember, however, that kids are growing up in the "fast food" generation. If they reject what you offer ask them for suggestions of what they want to eat and start from there.

Instead of accepting the idea that children hate vegetables try to find out which ones your children like. For example, most kids like corn on the cob and enjoy baked potatoes served with salsa.

Also, before you give up on feeding them any healthy foods, find out if there is a particular way that they like certain foods prepared. For example, some children do not like baked potatoes, but they do like mashed potatoes. This will provide some common "food ground" on which you and your children can build.

Listen carefully when your child expresses delight about certain sauces, colors or textures. Keep these in mind when planning your meals. For example, some children object to the soft texture of cooked mushrooms but many children love the bright red, slightly sweet taste of tomato sauce or ketchup.

Do not deny your children burgers on buns with ketchup, lettuce and all the trimmings. Try some of the wide array of meat-substitute products available at natural food stores, like burgers made from grains, tofu and other plant-derived sources. Buy several varieties and let your children decide which they like best. Then, serve on a wholesome bun with your favorite toppings.

Better yet, make your own inexpensive, nutritious, grain-based burgers using the directions in the recipe section. You can make up a large batch and store a dozen in your freezer ready to pop into the toaster oven for an instant lunch or dinner for a hungry child.

Stock up on other healthy "fast foods" that kids love like tofu hot dogs and vegetarian-style pizzas with soy cheese instead of dairy cheese. (A can of vegetarian-style chili or baked beans tastes great with tofu dogs!)

Learn to make a variety of sauces such as brown miso dressing or creamy white sauce. You will be amazed at how your children will consume green and yellow vegetables or a new grainloaf if they are covered with a favorite sauce.

Bring children into the kitchen, even at the toddler stage, and involve them in food preparation. Even a three year old can spread almond butter on bread and an older child can help prepare meals. The kitchen is a great place for them to learn responsibility, including kitchen safety (the first lesson) and "carry through" (cleaning up as you go).

Involve your children in your "smart" shopping trips so they begin to learn about and appreciate where their food comes from. Have them read the labels to you or introduce them to the farmers at the farmer's market, etc.

Find a place in the yard or even a window box and have your children grow some of their own food. Carrots and radishes are especially good choices as they grow quickly. A simple place to start is growing sprouts in a big jar in the kitchen. They will be excited with the quick results.

When introducing a new dish also prepare an "old reliable" recipe so that you can feel confident that your child will eat something. Oven fried or baked potatoes and corn kernels or on-the-cob are perennial favorites to have on the plate if your spinach lasagna meets with a rebellious "no!" from your child.

Kids love pasta and it is an excellent source of energy and protein. Serve whole-grain spaghetti and other noodle dishes with favorite sauces like tomato, pesto, garlic or extra virgin olive oil.

For very young children mix or purée foods in the blender with applesauce. Its sweet taste and pleasant texture will help a multitude of new foods slip into little stomachs.

Give children information that certain foods will help them grow: grains and beans build strong muscles, the calcium in greens builds strong bones and so on.

Buy tasty nut butters like almond and cashew. A tablespoon of these butters can not only be spread on bread but can also be mixed into fruit smoothies or used as a binder for grain burgers.

Purchase a good juice extractor and start making delicious fresh fruit and vegetable juices. Encourage your kids to help so they begin to realize that orange juice does not really come from a frozen can!

Make sure that your children have a source of vitamin B-12 in their diets *almost every day* to ensure normal growth. A great source is Super Blue-Green Algae. This is delicious in a banana smoothie. Vitamin B-12 is found in fortified breakfast cereals, breads and, of course, in multivitamins.

Children should never be forced to eat foods at mealtime. If they are not hungry do not start a civil war. Simply show children that you are putting their food in the refrigerator and they can eat it whenever they are hungry. Do not worry, Mother Nature will not let them starve!

Never hesitate to experiment along with your children to create new and interesting recipes.

Part II

Recipe Collection

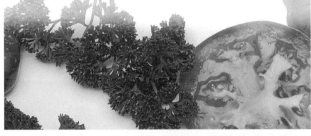

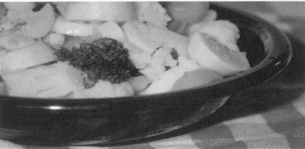

Breakfasts

Breakfast has always been my favorite meal. During the warm months I enjoy eating the delicious fresh fruits of the season: juicy nectarines, peaches, apricots, sweet strawberries, succulent melons and refreshing seedless grapes. I sometimes make a fruit bowl from some of these fruits and top it with a blended banana and a sweet fruit. Sometimes I blend it all up and make a simple, but delicious, thick fruit smoothie.

During the cold months I enjoy having a heartier breakfast of fruit and whole grains. My favorite and simplest way to do this is to take out my crockpot the night before and put in three grains like barley, brown rice and whole wheat berries and add water. When I wake up in the morning a wonderful pot of steaming whole grains awaits me. I will add some cinnamon and serve it with fruit and sometimes soy milk.

For special breakfasts, or on weekends, I will make scrambled tofu with fresh salsa and serve it with hashbrowns, or pancakes with spicy apple glaze.

I like to have some organic, whole grain boxed cereals and/or granola in my pantry so that I can enjoy a quick, tasty breakfast in the morning or any other time of the day.

Breakfasts can be very easy to prepare, delicious and nourishing. Start your eating day off right!

LF Paulette's Oil-Free Granola

3 cups oatmeal
1 cup wheat flakes
1 cup rye flakes
$1/2$ cup raisins
$1/2$ cup chopped dried apricots
$1/2$ cup chopped dates
1 cup chopped dried apples
$1/2$ cup raw sunflower seeds
$1/2$ cup rice syrup or maple syrup
$1/2$ cup hot water
1 T vanilla

Combine all dry ingredients, fruits and nuts in a large bowl. In another bowl mix the syrup, hot water and vanilla. Add to dry ingredients and mix well. Spread a $1/2$ inch layer on baking dishes and bake at 275°F for $1/2$ hour stirring occasionally. Remove from oven, let cool. Store in covered containers.

Helpful hints: Nuts may be omitted: use more wheat or rye flakes. Other dried fruits may be substituted for ones suggested. Be sure to stir every 20 minutes or so to keep the granola from sticking or burning.

VLF Fruit French Toast

SERVES 2 TO 4

> 1 banana, peeled
> 4 large strawberries, fresh or frozen
> ⅓ cup apple juice
> ½ t cinnamon
> 4 slices whole wheat bread

Blend together first four ingredients. Soak bread in the fruit mixture. Cook on both sides on lightly oiled or non-stick griddle until just beginning to brown.

LF Paulette's Pancakes

> ½ cup unbleached white flour
> ½ cup whole wheat pastry flour
> 1 T maple syrup
> pinch of salt
> pinch of cinnamon
> 1 cup soy milk (1% or non-fat) or rice milk
> 1 t lecithin oil
> ½-¾ cup chopped fresh fruit (eg. peaches, strawberries, banana)
> 1 T applesauce

Mix dry ingredients together. Mix wet ingredients together. Combine and add fruit stirring until the mixture is gooey. Drip by spoonful on oiled frying pan. Fry on both sides.

VLF Multi-Grain Waffles

SERVES 4 TO 6

> 3 cups water
> 2 cups rolled oats
> ½ cup rolled wheat

½ cup rolled rye
½ cup soy flour
2 T maple syrup

Blend all ingredients in blender until smooth. Let batter sit for about 5 minutes before spooning it into the hot waffle iron. Be sure batter is not too thick; a little thin is better than too thick.

VLF Blueberry Syrup

SERVES 6

3 cups unsweetened grape juice
3-4 T arrowroot powder or cornstarch
2 cups fresh or frozen blueberries
⅛ t lemon juice

Combine juices and thickeners in saucepan. Cook until thickened. Sauce should be thin like a syrup. If it gets too thick add more grape juice. Add blueberries. Serve warm or hot. Good over waffles, pancakes and french toast. You can blend the blueberries and add to thickened juice, but you will need more thickener.

VLF Spicy Apple Syrup

SERVES 4

1½ cups apple juice
1 T arrowroot powder or cornstarch
2 T lemon juice
⅛ t cinnamon

Bring to boil, stirring constantly until clear and thick.

TT Coconut-Flax Butter

This is delicious on toast and a great substitute for butter or margarine. Try it, but do not get hooked: it is still 100% fat. The following recipe is from Omega Nutrition.

1 cup unrefined coconut butter
½ cup fresh pressed, unrefined flaxseed oil

Freeze the flaxseed oil for at least two hours. Melt the coconut butter at low heat. Remove from heat and add frozen flaxseed oil. Mix and store in the refrigerator for up to six weeks.

VLF Apple Raisin Spice Muffins

MAKES 1 DOZEN

> 1 cup unbleached white flour
> 2 cups whole wheat pastry flour
> 1 t baking powder
> 1/2 t baking soda
> 1 t cinnamon
> 1/4 t nutmeg
> 1/2 t allspice
> 1 cup water
> 1/3 cup maple syrup or molasses
> 2 apples, cored and finely chopped
> 1/2 cup raisins

Preheat oven to 400° F degrees. Mix all the ingredients together in a large bowl. Pour batter into lightly oiled muffin tins. Bake for 20 minutes at 400° F.

VLF Whole Oats, Barley and Rice

SERVES 3

> 1/2 cup cut oats
> 1/2 cup whole barley
> 1/2 cup rice
> 3 cups water

Mix all together and steam for 1 hour. Serve with apple syrup.

VLF Hash Brown Potatoes

Shred raw scrubbed potatoes. Bake either on a teflon griddle or a waffle iron lightly sprayed with Pam. Crispness is determined by the amount you put into the waffle iron or on the griddle. Season with salt, onion and garlic or grated onion and paprika, or taco seasoning. Serve with ketchup.

VLF Yummy Granola

MAKES 9 CUPS

> 8 cups rolled oats (rolled rye or barley may
>   be substituted for 2 cups of oats)
> 1/2 cup cornmeal
> 2 ripe bananas

1 cup chopped dates
$^1/_2$ cup water
1 T vanilla

Combine oats and cornmeal in large bowl. Whiz fruit, water and vanilla in a blender, then add to the oats and cornmeal. Mix well. Spread $^1/_2$ inch thick on cookie sheets. Bake at 275°F approximately 90 minutes stirring every 30 minutes until golden and dry. If not quite dry turn oven off and leave pans in oven to complete drying. Store in airtight container

VLF Simple Oatmeal with Fresh Applesauce

SERVES 2

Version One:

$^1/_2$-$^3/_4$ cup water or apple juice
1 cup rolled oats
$^1/_4$ cup organic raisins
$^1/_2$ t cinnamon

Pour water or juice into a saucepan and bring to a boil. Add oatmeal, raisins and cinnamon and stir. Cover, turn off the element and let sit for 5 minutes. Serve mixed with fresh applesauce.

Version Two:

Same ingredients as above.

Mix all the ingredients together the night before, cover and let sit until morning. Serve mixed with fresh applesauce.

VLF Fresh Applesauce

3 apples (any good eating apple)
$^1/_4$ cup soaked organic raisins with $^1/_2$ cup raisin water
  (soak overnight)
$^1/_2$ t cinnamon
3 fresh strawberries

Cut up apples into big pieces. Peel the apples if they are not organic. Blend all the ingredients in a food processor until sauce consistency. Also, delicious as a dessert.

Salads and Sandwiches

How I used to love a tuna or chicken salad sandwich! Well those days are long gone but not at the expense of my enjoyment of a good, filling sandwich. Had I not changed my eating habits it is unlikely that I ever would have found out about using bean spreads (like hummus) or tofu cutlets in my sandwiches along with a good mustard, tomato slices and sprouts on wholegrain breads (like whole-wheat, rye, or multi-grain).

Pita pocket breads and flat breads like Mexican tortillas, East Indian chapatis and Armenian lavash add a whole new dimension to sandwich making because of their versatility in holding the ingredients. These are absolutely delicious and you are only limited by your own imagination. I have provided a number of ideas at the end of this section.

It is healthful to eat salads all year round but especially in the warm weather months do take advantage of the abundance of beautiful fresh and ideally organic produce that is available to you. Go ahead and experiment with fresh herbs. I tear up fresh basil and cilantro and just put it right into my salad bowl. Vary your salads and have more than one kind at a time. You can only benefit by eating fresh vitamin and mineral rich vegetables.

Eye appeal with salads is very important. Colors, shapes and textures can all be varied to spice up your salads. Try shredding, slicing, dicing and chopping your fruits and vegetables. If you have a food processor start using those attachments.

Do not forget about grain salads. This is an excellent way to use leftover cooked grains and make a complete meal. Grain salads are so tasty and full of nourishment. You can also use the leftover cooked grains in a sandwich wrap or in a pita pocket.

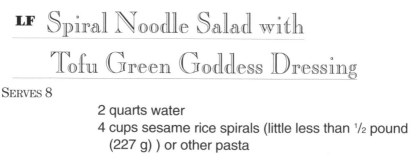

LF Spiral Noodle Salad with Tofu Green Goddess Dressing

SERVES 8

2 quarts water
4 cups sesame rice spirals (little less than 1/2 pound (227 g)) or other pasta
1/2 cup carrots, cut in thin half moon slices
1/2 cup cauliflower (or sunchoke), separated into

small florets, or diced
$^1/_2$ cup onion, diced
$^1/_2$ cup red cabbage, thinly sliced
$^1/_2$ cup sunflower seeds, toasted and sprinkled with
    natural soy sauce
$^1/_4$ cup parsley, chopped

Tofu Green Goddess Dressing:
MAKES 1$^1/_2$ CUPS

$^1/_2$ pound (227 g) tofu, soft and fresh (fat reduced)
2 T natural soy sauce
2 T rice vinegar
1 cup parsley, chopped
$^1/_4$ cup water

Bring water to boil and add pasta. Cook until done, about 10 minutes. Strain noodles, reserving hot cooking liquid, then run noodles under cold water, drain and set aside to cool. Return enough water to pot for use in boiling tofu for dressing.

Steam carrots and cauliflower until crispy-soft, about five-minutes, and remove to cool. Steam onion and red cabbage about 3 minutes and cool. Mix noodles and vegetables. Toss with seeds and parsley just before serving to retain crisp textures.

To prepare Tofu Green Goddess Dressing boil tofu 5 minutes, drain and allow to cool. Blend remaining ingredients then crumble in tofu and blend until creamy smooth. For large amounts start with no water and add it as needed.

Pour dressing over salad and serve on the side.

VLF Pasta Salad

SERVES 8 TO 10

1 t salt
12 ounces pasta shells (about 2 cups)
1 cup artichoke hearts, quartered
1 cup button mushrooms, quartered
2 T lemon juice
$^1/_4$ cup cider vinegar
2 t prepared mustard
$^1/_4$ cup chopped green onions
$^1/_2$ t each: basil, oregano, black pepper

¹/₂ t salt
1 garlic clove
3 T water
2 green onions, chopped (include greens)
3 T fresh parsley, chopped
1 small red bell pepper, diced

Bring water to a boil in a large kettle then add salt and pasta. Cook pasta until just tender – al dente (six to twelve minutes, depending on type of pasta used). Rinse, drain and place into a large bowl. Add the quartered artichoke hearts and mushrooms.

In a blender combine the lemon juice, vinegar, mustard, green onions, seasonings and water. Process until smooth. Pour over pasta and allow to marinate until pasta is cool.

Add green onions, parsley, and red bell pepper and gently toss to mix.

VLF Cucumber Salad
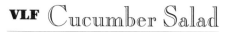

SERVES 4

Simple and delicious, especially in the summertime when tomatoes and cucumbers are in season.

3 large cucumbers, peeled if they are waxed
2 large tomatoes
¹/₂ small red onion
¹/₂ t basil or 1 t fresh if available
¹/₂ t dill weed or 1 t fresh if available
1 T chopped fresh parsley
apple cider vinegar or lemon juice

Slice the cucumbers in half lengthwise and scoop out the seeds. Cut into bite-sized pieces. Dice the tomatoes, and chop the red onion fairly finely. Toss the vegetables together, then sprinkle with basil, dill and fresh parsley. Add enough vinegar to coat all the vegetables and toss. Chill before serving if possible.

VLF Aztec Salad

SERVES 10

This salad is full of color and taste and keeps well.

1¹/₂ cups dry black beans
3¹/₂ cups water

2 cups frozen corn, thawed
2 large tomatoes, diced
1 large green bell pepper, diced
1 large red or yellow bell pepper, diced
$1/2$ t crushed red pepper or a pinch of cayenne
$1/2$ cup chopped red onion
$3/4$ cup chopped fresh cilantro (optional)

Dressing ingredients:

2 T apple cider vinegar
2 garlic cloves, minced
2 t cumin
1 t coriander
$1/2$-1 t salt
juice of one lime or lemon

Wash beans, soak overnight, spill off soaking water then combine with water and simmer until tender, 2 – 3 hours. Drain and cool.

In a large bowl, combine beans, corn, tomatoes, bell peppers, crushed red pepper, red onion and fresh cilantro.

Whisk together dressing ingredients and pour over salad. Toss gently to mix.

LF Chinese Cabbage Noodle Salad

SERVES 4 TO 6

This is a recipe that I make over and over again because it tastes great and is a fabulous way to eat raw cabbage with all its powerful nutrient value.

$1/2$ large head or one small head of cabbage, thinly sliced
4 green onions, chopped
$1^1/2$-2 T minced cilantro
2 pkgs. top ramen from natural food store
2 T sesame seeds. toasted
$1/4$ cup sliced almonds, toasted

Dressing:

$1/2$ cup seasoned rice vinegar
$1/2$ cup water
1 T toasted sesame oil
1 t tamari
1 t sweetener such as maple syrup

In a large bowl combine cabbage, onions and cilantro. Crumble top ramen noodles into mixture and sprinkle with the seasonings packet that comes with it. Toast the sesame seeds and the almonds in a dry skillet over a medium flame until slightly browned. Blend all the dressing ingredients together then pour over the cabbage mixture and stir. Let sit for 30-60 minutes until the noodles are soft. Add the seeds and nuts last so that they remain crunchy.

LF Barley Salad

SERVES 5

> 1/3 cup barley
> 2 T vegetarian broth powder
> 1 cup water
> 1/2 cup green pepper, chopped fine
> 1/4 t dill weed
> 1/2 t parsley
> juice of one lemon, more or less to taste
> 1 cup carrots, quartered, thinly sliced and raw
> 1/4 t onion salt
> 1 T Nayonaise (made from tofu, found in natural
> food store)
> dash of minced garlic

Cook the barley in the broth and water for 45 minutes. All the water should be absorbed. You may have to add just a bit more. When cool add the remaining ingredients. Mix all ingredients and serve on a bed of lettuce and chopped tomatoes.

VLF Marinated Vegetable Salad

SERVES 5

> 3/4 cup fresh lemon juice
> 4 medium dates
> 1 medium head cauliflower, cut into small florets
> 4 medium zucchini, halved and sliced
> 1 cup cherry tomatoes, halved (may use other tomatoes)
> 1/2 cup chopped green pepper
> 1 T fresh basil or 1 t dried basil
> 1 t salt

Blend the dates with the lemon juice and combine with all the other ingredients in a covered bowl which can be turned upside down occasionally to distribute the dressing. Refrigerate overnight. Will be good for up to three days.

TT Eggless Tofu Salad

1 pkg. tofu (16 ounces)
¼ cup mayonnaise (eggless)
1 t flaxseed oil or Omega's Essential Blend
1T dijon mustard
½ t tumeric
2 celery stalks, chopped
1-2 scallions, chopped
¼ cup diced dill pickle
2 T nutritional yeast
salt to taste

Using a fork or potato masher, mash the tofu until it is the consistency of chopped hard boiled egg. Add remaining ingredients and mix well. Serve as a sandwich spread or dip.

VLF Chickpea Italiana

SERVES 4

1 15-ounce (425-ml) can chickpeas (garbanzo beans), drained and mashed
¼ t oregano
⅛ t pepper
¼ t onion powder
4 T tomato sauce

Mash all the ingredients together in a bowl with fork. Serve on whole wheat bread with lettuce.

LF Chickpea Paté (Hummus)

SERVES 4

Serve as a dip or a sandwich spread.

1 15-ounce (425-ml) can chickpeas (garbanzo beans) or
2 cups cooked chickpeas (organic if possible)
1-2 garlic cloves, minced
¼ cup tahini (sesame seed butter)
2 T lemon juice
¼ t salt
1 T finely chopped parsley
¼ t each cumin and paprika

Drain the beans, reserving the liquid. Mash beans then add remaining ingredients and mix well. If mixture is too dry add enough of the reserved bean liquid to achieve the desired consistency.

ᴛᴛ Veggie Paté

MAKES A 9-INCH SQUARE CAKE

This recipe comes from a wonderful little recipe collection book produced by a Toronto vegetarian society called Vegetarian Tastes of Toronto. It can be served with crackers, used as a sandwich filler or used to stuff celery. This paté keeps in the refrigerator for several days or can be frozen.

> 1¹/₂ cups sunflower seeds, ground
> ¹/₂ cup whole wheat flour
> ¹/₂ cup nutritional yeast
> 2 T lemon juice
> 1 raw potato, grated
> 4 green onions, sliced
> 1 stalk of celery, grated
> 1 carrot, grated
> 1 T oil
> ³/₄ cup warm water
> 1 T or more of each, thyme, basil, sage, salt and pepper

Grind the sunflower seeds in a blender. Mix all the ingredients together. Press into a 9-inch square pan and bake at 350ºF for 1 hour until golden brown. Let cool.

ᴠʟꜰ Bean Burgers

SERVES 8

> 1 cup baked beans or seasoned cooked beans
> ¹/₂ cup bread crumbs or mashed potatoes
> 1 onion, finely chopped
> 2 carrots, finely grated
> ¹/₂ t sage
> tomato sauce to moisten
> salt to taste

Mix all ingredients together and shape into patties. Brown on teflon griddle and serve with tomato sauce or home-made ketchup.

VLF Legume Spread

> 3 cups kidney beans (cooked or canned)
> 3 cups chickpeas (garbanzo beans) (cooked or canned)
> 1 cup celery, finely chopped
> 1 cup onion, finely chopped
> 1 T dill weed
> 1/2 cup pimento
> 1/2 cup green pepper
> 1 T fresh parsley

Blend in food processor with just enough juice from beans to make a thick spread. Add remaining ingredients and mix well.

VLF Chickpea Spread

> 1 cup chickpeas (garbanzo beans), drained
> 1/4 cup green onions, finely chopped
> 1 small garlic clove, minced
> 1 T fresh parsley
> 1/4 cup celery
> 1 T nutritional yeast
> 1/2 t sweet basil
> 1/2 cup green pepper, finely chopped
> 1/4 cup pimento

Blend in food processor or blender with enough water to make a thick spread.

TT Date-Banana-Almond Butter Spread

SERVES 4

This spread is delicious and much lower in fat and higher in nutrition than peanut butter. Children and adults love it!

> 1 banana
> 1/4 cup almond butter
> 5 pitted dates, chopped

Pulse in a food processor until blended.

Sandwich Wrap Ideas

Use whole-wheat chapatis or vegetarian tortillas or best yet Lavash bread (no added oil) which has a long oval shape and is found in Middle Eastern stores. Cut into 4 to 6 rectangles. Use one piece, spread mustard or other condiment on, place filling at one end with sprouts, tomatoes, cucumbers, lettuce or red peppers and roll up. Try the following wonderful fillings. Some of them can be found readily in the deli section of your natural food store, or better yet make your own from the recipes in this book.

Aztec Salad* with brown rice

Chickpea Spread* or Hummus

Broiled or Baked Tofu

Tofu Teriyaki* and brown rice

Veggie Paté* and salad

Spanish Rice* with Refried Beans*

Legume Spread* with Cucumber Salad*

Bulgur Wheat Salad* (Tabouli) with Cucumber Salad*

Barley Salad* with Marinated Vegetable Salad*

Lentil Dal* with millet

Chickpea Italiana* with Marinated Vegetable Salad*

Mediterranean Oven "Fries"* and steamed veggies

leftover Chili Beans* with rice and Easy Salsa*

crumbled veggie burger with salad

* Recipe in Recipe Collection

Soups

Soups have always been associated with nourishment and comfort. When I was growing up, if I was sick, my mother would cook up a big pot of chicken soup. Today if I or my family are feeling a little under the weather, I will make a pot of miso or vegetable soup. Miso soup has the same soothing effect that chicken soup used to have for me but it is considerably healthier.

Having some homemade vegetable stock on hand will make your soups richer and tastier. However, do not let a lack of it keep you from creating a delicious soup. Miso and vegetable broth powders and brown mushrooms can add a lot of depth and taste to your soups. Soy milks, nut milks and rice milk can be used for creamy soups.

When I open my refrigerator door and notice that many of my vegetables are less than fresh, I know it is time to make soup. A hearty soup, like a Lentil soup or corn chowder, with a piece of dark, wholesome bread is one of my favorite winter meals.

VLF Paulette's Vegetable-Nori Soup

SERVES 5

Sauté:

1 large onion, chopped
2 celery stalks
2 carrots
8 ounces (227 ml) mushrooms
$^1/_2$ cup water
1 T Bragg Liquid Aminos or natural soy sauce
1 T vegetarian broth powder

Add:

1 cup red cabbage, chopped
$^2/_3$ cup nori pieces, rinsed
$^3/_4$ cup leeks, sliced
1 cup green cabbage, chopped
1 red pepper, chopped
1$^1/_2$ cups green beans, kale or spinach
1 t thyme
1 bunch fresh parsley, chopped
2 t cumin

2 t basil
2 t oregano
3 T vegetarian broth powder
dash cayenne

Add water to cover vegetables, parsley, seasonings. Add 3 T Bragg Liquid Aminos or tamari.Cover. Simmer 1 hour. Add 3 cubed potatoes. Simmer another ½ hour.

VLF Minestrone

SERVES 8

1 small onion, chopped
1 clove garlic, minced
1 t extra virgin olive oil
3 cups tomato juice
3 cups water
2 carrots, diced
1 celery stalk, diced
2 medium potatoes, diced
1 T parsley, chopped
1 t salt
1 t basil
1 medium zucchini, diced
½ cup pasta shells
1 cup cooked kidney beans or 1 15-ounce (425-ml) can, drained
2½ cups chopped greens (spinach, collards, romaine, etc.)

Sauté onion and garlic in olive oil until soft and golden. Add tomato juice, water, carrots, celery, potatoes, parsley, salt and basil. Bring to a simmer then cover and cook 20 minutes.

Add remaining ingredients then cover and simmer an additional 20-30 minutes. Additional tomato juice or water may be added if the soup is too thick.

VLF Split Pea Soup

SERVES 8

2 cups split peas, rinsed
5 cups hot water
1 cup carrots, sliced and diced

1 cup celery, sliced
1 medium onion, chopped
2 cloves garlic, minced
$\frac{1}{2}$ t marjoram
$\frac{1}{2}$ t basil
$\frac{1}{4}$ t cumin
1$\frac{1}{2}$ t salt
$\frac{1}{4}$ t black pepper
pinch cayenne

Rinse split peas, then place them in a large kettle with the remaining ingredients. Bring to a simmer, then cover loosely and cook until the peas are tender, 1-2 hours.

Crockpot method: Place all ingredients in a crockpot. Cover and cook on "High" for 3-4 hours, until the peas are soft and the vegetables are tender.

VLF Green Velvet Soup

SERVES 8

1 onion, chopped
2 celery stalks, sliced
2 potatoes, scrubbed and diced
$\frac{3}{4}$ cup split peas, rinsed
2 bay leaves
6 cups water or stock
2 medium zucchini, diced
1 medium broccoli stalk, chopped
1 bunch fresh spinach, washed and chopped
1$\frac{1}{2}$ t salt
$\frac{1}{2}$ t basil
$\frac{1}{4}$ t black pepper
pinch cayenne

Place onion, celery, potatoes, split peas and bay leaves in a large kettle with water or stock and bring to a boil. Lower heat, cover and simmer 1 hour. Remove bay leaves.

Add zucchini, broccoli, spinach and seasonings and simmer 20 minutes. Transfer to a blender in several small batches and blend until smooth, holding the lid on tightly. Return to kettle and heat until steamy.

Crockpot version: Place all ingredients into a crockpot and cook on "High" for 4-5 hours. Purée as above and serve immediately.

VLF Lentil Soup with Elbow Macaroni

SERVES 8

¹/₄ cup vegetarian broth powder
2 garlic cloves
1 large red onion, finely chopped
1 bay leaf
1 large celery stalk, finely chopped
1 medium carrot, finely chopped
1¹/₂ cups brown or green lentils, washed and cleaned
3 sprigs fresh thyme or ¹/₂ t dried
¹/₂ cup fresh parsley, minced
14 cups water
6 fresh plum tomatoes, peeled, seeded, chopped and
    juice squeezed out and reserved; or 1 16-ounce (454-ml)
    can plum tomatoes, seeds squeezed out, tomatoes
    chopped and juice reserved (optional)
¹/₂ cup elbow macaroni or other similar pasta
2 T soy miso (optional)
ground rock salt
fresh ground pepper

Heat vegetable broth with garlic and red onion in a soup pot. Add bay leaf, celery and carrot and sauté briefly. Add lentils, mixing well. Add thyme and parsley and mix in. Cook on medium heat until vegetables begin to soften slightly then add water, juice from tomatoes and chopped tomatoes. Bring to a boil, cover and simmer for 45 minutes.

Stir in pasta and miso. Return to a boil and simmer, uncovered, for 30 minutes longer or until pasta is tender. Add extra water to thin the soup, if necessary, then season with salt and pepper to taste.

LF Traditional Ukrainian Cabbage Soup

SERVES 10 TO 12

1 T extra virgin olive oil
2 cups sliced leeks
1 medium red onion, sliced
2 carrots, halved and cut in ¹/₈-inch rounds
1 medium green cabbage, coarsely chopped (7–8 cups)
1 t dried thyme
7 cups boiling water

1 T vegetarian broth powder (optional)
1 heaping T light miso or 1 vegetable broth cube
3 T lemon juice
1 T rice syrup
2 cups or 2 medium tomatoes, peeled and chopped
freshly ground pepper

Heat oil, leeks, and onion in a pot. Sauté stirring for 2 minutes or until vegetables begin to soften. Add carrots and cabbage and continue sautéing over medium heat until cabbage begins to wilt. Add thyme and stir well.

Add boiling water and broth to vegetables. Stir well. Cover and bring to a boil and simmer over medium heat for 10 minutes. Remove cover and stir in miso, lemon juice and rice syrup. Simmer for 3 or 4 minutes longer then stir in tomatoes. Add ground black pepper to taste.

LF Corn Chowder

SERVES 5

1 onion, chopped
2 T water
2 cups water
2 celery stalks, chopped
2 carrots, chopped
2 17-ounce (483-ml) cans creamed corn (non-dairy)
1 cup soy milk (1% or non-fat)
1 potato, chopped
2 large garlic cloves, minced
1/4 t nutmeg
salt and pepper to taste

Sauté onion in 2 T water medium-high heat until soft. Add rest of water and chopped celery and carrots. Cook 10 minutes. Add creamed corn, soy milk, chopped potato and spices. Continue cooking for another 10 minutes. Serve hot.

VLF My Favorite Borscht

SERVES 8 TO 10

This is a wonderful soup for a cold day winter day. It is also a great liver cleanser. This soup freezes well.

2 large onions, chopped

1 cup carrots, sliced
4 cups green cabbage, sliced
1¹/₂ cups beets, cubed
2 cups potatoes
¹/₄ cup tamari or natural soy sauce
6 cups vegetable stock
2 bay leaves
2 T parsley, chopped
1 t salt
cayenne pepper to taste
juice of 1 large lemon
1 T maple syrup or other natural sweetener
1 cup fresh tomatoes, peeled and chopped

Sauté the onions and carrots in a little stock. Add the sliced cabbage, beets, potatoes and soy sauce. Add the stock, bay leaves and all seasonings. Let come to a boil, reduce heat, add lemon juice and sweetener. Let the soup cook on low heat for ¹/₂ hour and then add the chopped tomatoes. Cook for another ¹/₂ hour.

Main Dishes

The recipes I chose for this section of the book were selected with three important criteria: ease of preparation, taste and common ingredients. Many of these recipes call for the use of legumes.

About Legumes

The term legumes is not commonly used but is the broad category that includes beans, lentils, black-eyed peas, split peas and even peanuts. The enormous variety of legumes and the endless ways to prepare them make them an excellent source of high-quality protein. In addition, unlike animal protein, they also provide fiber and complex carbohydrates.

Shopping for legumes is easy. They are extremely economical and available in the supermarkets and natural food stores in packages and in bulk. Legumes store very well and will keep in an air-tight glass jar for up to a year.

Since legumes freeze very well, it is a good idea to double your bean recipes and freeze some to be used at a later date. You can find canned beans (in lead-free cans) at the natural food store as well as beans packed in glass jars. Using these dramatically cuts down on your food preparation time and does not significantly alter the end result. Another quick easy option is to use packaged bean flakes that you reconstitute with water.

Beans and Digestion

There are a number of things you can do to decrease any discomfort and gas you may experience in digesting beans.

1. Before cooking the beans, soak them overnight and in the morning discard the soaking water: this process greatly reduces the complex sugars that may cause gas.

2. Savory and the sea vegetable, kombu, may be added to the cooking liquid to enhance digestibility.

3. Do not add salt to the cooking process as this toughens the beans. Add salt at the end.

TT Jeff's Favorite "Neat" Loaf

SERVES 8 TO 10

> 1 large onion, chopped
> 2 celery stalks, chopped

1 15-ounce (425-ml) can chickpeas (garbanzo beans),
   drained and mashed well
$1/2$ cup walnuts, ground
$1/3$ cup wheat germ
1 pound (454 g) frozen tofu, defrosted, squeezed dry and
   crumbled
2 T tomato paste
2 T miso
1-2 T natural soy sauce
$1/2$ t allspice
1 t thyme
$1/2$ t chervil
1 t oregano
freshly ground pepper to taste
3-4 T tahini mixed with a little water to make a thick paste

Topping:
$1/3$ cup ketchup
2 T natural soy sauce

Preheat the oven to 350°F. Sauté the onions and celery in a little oil or water until tender. Combine all the ingredients and pat into a greased loaf pan. Combine the topping ingredients and smear on top of the loaf. Bake for 1 hour. Turn off the heat and allow to sit in the oven for an additional 20 – 30 minutes or at room temperature for 15 minutes before unmolding and slicing or it may not hold together well. Serve with gravy.

TT Tofu Loaf

SERVES 16

A great leftover for sandwiches.

2 garlic cloves, diced
1 onion, diced
1 carrot, diced
1 red pepper, diced
1 celery stalk, diced
2 T tamari
2 pounds (908 g) firm tofu, mashed
4 slices whole-wheat bread
1 T oil
1 T tamari
1 garlic clove, minced

³/₄ cup nutritional yeast
2 T tahini mixed with 2 T water
2 t basil
2 t oregano
¹/₂ t turmeric
¹/₄ cup vegetarian broth powder (1 T powder mixed with ¹/₄ cup water)

Heat 5 T of water in a medium skillet; add garlic, onion, pepper, carrot, and celery. Season with 1 T tamari. When vegetables are tender, remove from heat and put in medium bowl, add mashed tofu. Cut bread into small crouton-sized pieces; quick fry with oil, 1 T tamari, 1 garlic clove, and 3/4 cup nutritional yeast. Add bread to tofu mixture, and season with remaining ingredients. Combine well. Place mixture into a nonstick casserole; bake at 3500F for 35 minutes.

Allow to cool; slide a butter knife along the sides then turn upside-down on a plate to remove from casserole. Serve with gravy.

VLF Polenta Squares with Red Vegetable Sauce

SERVES 16

Polenta:
    2 cups cornmeal or flour
    6 cups water
    1 T natural soy sauce or ¹/₂ t sea salt.

Italian Red Sauce: makes 2¹/₂ cups
    4 cups or 1 pound (454 g) carrots (or winter squash or pumpkin)
    1 medium beet
    ¹/₂ cup water
    1 bay leaf
    1 t each oregano and basil
    2 T natural soy sauce, sauerkraut juice or miso

Red Vegetable Sauce:
    ¹/₄ cup water
    1 onion, thinly sliced
    3 cups broccoli, cut in 2 inch lengths, then in ¹/₄ inch strips lengthwise, keeping florets intact

To make polenta, bring ingredients to boil then simmer uncovered for one hour. Stir about every 10 minutes. Pour hot cornmeal mush into standard 8-inch square baking dish to set, about one hour at room temperature.

To make the Italian Red Sauce place vegetables in a pressure cooker with water and bay leaf. Bring to pressure then turn heat to medium-low and time for five minutes. Discard bay leaf and purée ingredients with seasonings and soy sauce in blender. Use miso only if you are not serving it in another dish at the meal.

To prepare the Red Vegetable Sauce, place water, onion and broccoli in saucepan and bring to boil. Simmer covered until done, about 10 minutes.

To assemble dish, cut gelled polenta into 16 squares. Top each square with a little onion and broccoli and a dollop of the sauce.

For large volumes of this recipe simply multiply ingredients.

ᴛᴛ Millet "Mashed Potatoes"

Serves 4

Millet is such a versatile undervalued grain. Try this way of preparing it.

> 1 T sunflower oil (or other kind)
> 1 onion, coarsely chopped
> 1 cup millet
> 2 cups cauliflower, about $1/2$ pound (227 g)
> 2-$2^1/2$ cups water, less for pressure cooking, more for
>   boiling
> $1/2$ t sea salt

Rinse and drain millet. In pressure cooker or pot, heat oil and sauté onion briefly. Add millet and continue to sauté. Add remaining ingredients, cover, and bring to pressure or boil. Turn heat low to pressure cook for 15 minutes or boil for $1/2$ hour. No flame spreader needed.

When millet is done, while still hot, purée mixture in food processor or Foley food mill (also known as ricer) until smooth, or mash ingredients well. Transfer to serving bowl and allow to sit for about 10-15 minutes before serving for texture to firm up to proper consistency. Serve with Country Gravy* poured over or at the side.

Variation: Millet "Mashed Potato" Casserole.

Preheat oven to 350ᵒF Prepare as above reserving 1 t oil, then transfer mixture to corn-oiled pie pan or casserole dish and smooth surface. Mix remaining 1 t oil with 1 T soy sauce and drizzle it over top. Bake for $1/2$ hour. Let sit 15 minutes before serving.

* Recipe in Recipe Collection

VLF Tomato-Lentil Stew

SERVES 6 TO 8

> 2 cups uncooked lentils
> 1 cup onion, chopped
> $^1/_2$ cup celery, sliced
> $^1/_2$ cup carrot, diced
> 4 cups tomato juice
> 1 T parsley, dried
> $^1/_2$ t cumin
> 1 t oregano
> 1 t sweet basil
> 1 t salt
> lemon juice to taste

Cook lentils, onion, carrot and celery together in 4 cups tomato juice for $^1/_2$ hour. Add other ingredients and simmer $^1/_2$ hour or until lentils are cooked. Delicious served over whole-wheat toast or brown rice.

LF Chili Beans

SERVES 8

Enjoy this chili with corn bread and salad or serve it over grains or pasta.

> 3 cups dried pinto beans
> 8-9 cups water
> 4 cloves garlic, minced
> 1 t cumin
> 2 onions, chopped
> 2 bell peppers, diced
> 1 T extra virgin olive oil
> 1 28-ounce (795-ml) can tomato sauce
> 2 cups corn, fresh or frozen
> 1 t salt
> 1$^1/_2$ t chili powder
> $^1/_8$ t cayenne
> fresh cilantro, chopped

Wash beans thoroughly, then soak overnight. Discard soaking water. Place beans in a large kettle with fresh water and cook them along with the garlic and cumin until they are tender, about 2$^1/_2$ hours. When the beans are tender, sauté the onion and bell pepper in olive oil until the onion is soft and golden, then add to the cooked beans, along with all remaining ingredients. Simmer at least 30 minutes.

Crockpot method: Begin cooking the beans in the morning, using hot water and the high setting on the crockpot. By mid to late afternoon the beans will be tender. Add the remaining ingredients (excluding oil) and continue cooking on high setting until dinner time.

LF Lasagna

SERVES 6

Delicious with a white sauce that satisfies the desire for dairy.

> 2^1/$_2$-3 cups Italian Red Sauce (recipe follows)
> 3 cups Italian White Sauce (recipe follows)
> ^{1}/$_2$ pound (227 g) whole-wheat lasagna noodles, broken in thirds
> 16 cups or 4 quarts water
> 2 T parsley, minced for garnish

Italian Red Sauce:

> 4 cups or 1 pound (454 g) carrots and/or winter squash, cut in 1-inch chunks
> 1 small beet, cut in 1-inch chunks
> ^{1}/$_2$ cup water
> 1 bay leaf
> 2 T natural soy sauce or miso or 3 T sauerkraut juice
> 1 t each oregano or basil

Italian White Sauce:

> 2 large onions, thinly sliced
> 1 T extra virgin olive oil
> 2 T water
> 4 large garlic cloves, finely sliced
> 1 pound (454 g) tofu, fresh (fat-reduced)
> 2 T natural soy sauce
> 1 t sea salt
> 1 T each oregano and basil

Carrots and/or sweet winter squashes such as sweetmeat or buttercup have the best flavors for the red sauce. (This is also a nice way to use pumpkin, but the flavor is milder.)

To prepare Italian Red Sauce, pressure cook vegetables in water with bay leaf for 5 minutes. Discard bay leaf and transfer ingredients to food processor, blender or food mill with soy sauce, salt and herbs. Purée until smooth. There is no need to remove the skin from soft-skinned squashes (or pumpkins), but do so for those with dark green or hard skins, after cooking. To double recipe, keep water at $\frac{1}{2}$ cup. For larger volumes, use 1 cup water.

To make Italian White Sauce, heat oil in a large skillet and sauté onions briefly. Add water and cook, stirring occasionally, until onions are almost soft, about 5 minutes. Add garlic, crumble tofu over garlic and add remaining ingredients. Cover to cook for about 5 minutes more. Purée ingredients until creamy smooth, or blend just half the mixture for a chunkier effect.

To cook noodles, in a large capacity pot (5 quart) bring water to a rolling boil, add noodles and boil until soft yet firm or al dente, about 15-29 minutes. Pour off water and run noodles under cool water. Drain and set aside until you are ready to assemble lasagna.

Preheat oven to 350⁰F.

To assemble lasagna, spread a little red sauce over the bottom of a standard 8 inch square baking dish. Layer one thickness of lasagna noodles over sauce, side-by-side, cutting off any extra from ends. Follow pasta with white sauce. Repeat this order (red sauce-pasta-white sauce-pasta) ending with red sauce. In all, there will be 4 layers of pasta, 3 of red sauce and 2 of white sauce.

Bake casserole for $\frac{1}{2}$ hour. Garnish with parsley to serve.

LF Simply Wonderful Vegetable Stew

SERVES 6 TO 8

Easy and wonderful. Serve with corn bread and salad.

> 2 medium onions, chopped
> 1$\frac{1}{2}$ t oil
> 1 28-ounce (795-ml) can Italian-style stewed tomatoes
> 2 garlic cloves, minced
> 1 large bell pepper, seeded and diced
> 6 medium red potatoes, unpeeled, cut into $\frac{1}{2}$-inch cubes
> 1 t each basil and oregano
> 1 t fine herbs (mixed Italian herbs)
> $\frac{1}{2}$ t salt
> 1-2 cups green peas, fresh or frozen

In a large kettle, sauté onion until soft and golden. Add all remaining ingredients except peas and bring to a simmer. Cover and cook 20-25 minutes, until potatoes are just tender. Stir in peas and continue cooking until heated through.

LF Vegetable Pot Pie

SERVES 8

Stock:

4 cups or 1 quart water
1 T natural soy sauce
1 t corn oil
1 t thyme

Vegetables:

1 onion
$^1/_2$ carrot
$^1/_2$ turnip, rutabaga or parsnip
$^1/_4$ green cabbage head
$^1/_2$ cup peas, if edible pod variety, cut in 1-inch slices
    (optional, in season)
1 cup wheat meat (seitan)

Gravy: makes a little more than 1 cup.

1 cup hot stock
$^1/_3$ cup whole-wheat pastry flour
2 T natural soy sauce

Top Cutout Crust:

$^1/_4$-$^1/_3$ cup warm stock, less if more oil
1-2 T extra virgin olive oil
$^1/_8$ t sea salt
$^3/_4$ cup whole-wheat pastry flour
$^1/_4$ cup corn flour or meal
$^1/_8$ t thyme

Bring stock ingredients to a boil. Preheat oven to 350°F.

Cut vegetables and wheat meat into 1-inch chunks. Add root vegetables to boiling stock and when boiling resumes turn heat down to slow-boil for 5 minutes. Add cabbage and peas and cook 5 minutes more. Strain out vegetables and measure stock.

To make gravy, return 1 cup hot stock to pot and add flour and soy sauce. Stir with wire whisk over high heat until mixture becomes smooth and thick, about 1-2 minutes. Pour gravy over vegetables, add wheat meat chunks and mix well. Transfer to lightly-oiled pie pan.

Make top crust by mixing warm stock, oil and salt, then adding to flour. Mix well, knead briefly to form a cohesive ball and roll out to a thin round. Sprinkle thyme over surface and press it in with a rolling pin. To make a decorative air vent, cut a hole in the center of the dough with a cookie cutter. Lay pastry on top of pie filling and tuck edges under all the way around. Poke holes on top only if you have not used the cookie cutter. Bake for ½ hour

For large amounts, increase ingredients proportionately.

Variation: Omit wheat meat and substitute another ½ carrot and turnip.

VLF 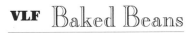 Baked Beans

SERVES 8

These beans are cooked in two stages: first the beans must be cooked until tender, then they are baked, in an oven or a crockpot, with the remaining ingredients. Either way, the longer they cook, the more wonderful they become.

> 2½ cups or 1 pound (454 g) navy beans
> 1 red onion, chopped
> 1 15-ounce (425-ml) can tomato sauce
> ½ cup molasses
> 2 t prepared mustard
> 2 T red wine vinegar
> 1 garlic clove, minced
> 1-2 t salt

Wash beans, then soak overnight. Discard soaking water. Place beans in a kettle and cover with water to 1 inch above beans. Simmer until tender, 2-3 hours. When tender, add all remaining ingredients. Transfer to an ovenproof dish and bake at 350°F for 2-3 hours.

Crockpot method: After soaking beans, place in a crockpot with water to 1 inch above beans. Cook on High until beans are tender. Add all remaining ingredients and continue cooking on High for 2-3 hours.

LF Dal

SERVES 6 TO 8

This dal is made with yellow split peas.

> 1½ cups yellow split peas
> 4 cups water
> 1 t salt
> 2 T safflower oil
> 1 t cumin seeds (or ground cumin)
> 1 t turmeric

1 small cinnamon stick
$\frac{1}{4}$ t cayenne
$\frac{1}{4}$ t ginger
$\frac{1}{4}$ t coriander
$\frac{1}{4}$ t mustard seeds

Wash the peas and place them in a kettle with the water and salt. Cover and simmer until tender, about 1 hour.

Heat oil in a skillet and add the spices to it. Cook and stir them a few minutes then remove the pan from the heat. Pour in the cooked peas being careful to protect yourself from the spattering which may occur. Return the pan to the heat and simmer, stirring often, until the dal is fairly thick. Serve very hot with curried rice or pilaf.

LF Lentil Dal

SERVES 8

2 large onions, chopped
4 garlic cloves, minced
$1\frac{1}{2}$ T oil
1 t salt
1 t turmeric
2 t cumin seeds
2 t coriander powder
1 t cayenne
2 cups lentils, rinsed
5-6 cups boiling water

In a heavy kettle, sauté the onions and garlic in oil until the onion starts to turn golden, then stir in the salt and spices and continue to cook another minute. Add the lentils and boiling water (start with 5 cups) then cover and simmer 1 hour, until the lentils are tender. Stir occasionally while cooking. If the mixture becomes too dry add more water.

LF Refried Beans

SERVES 6 TO 8

These tasty refried beans are made with much less fat than is used in more traditional recipes. Be sure to clean and wash the beans thoroughly before soaking and cooking.

$1\frac{1}{2}$ cups pinto beans, dried
4 cups water

> 2 garlic cloves, minced
> 1 t cumin
> ¹/₃ t cayenne
> 1 onion, chopped
> 1 T extra virgin olive oil
> 1 15-ounce can tomatoes, chopped with their juice
> ¹/₄ cup diced Anaheim chilis (such as Ortega brand chilis)
> ¹/₂ t salt

Pick the beans over, removing any stones or other debris. Wash thoroughly, then soak in 4 cups of water for 8 hours.

Discard water, rinse beans and place them in a kettle with 4 cups water, two garlic cloves, the cumin and cayenne. Simmer until tender, about 3 hours.

In a large skillet, sauté the onion and garlic in extra virgin olive oil until the onion is golden. Stir in the tomatoes and chilis then begin adding the beans, a cup at a time, mashing them as you add them. When all the beans have been added, stir to mix, then cook over low heat, stirring frequently, until the mixture is quite thick. Add salt to taste.

LF Pasta with Broccoli and Pine Nuts

SERVES 6 TO 8

Perfect for a light supper on a hot summer evening. Serve with a crisp green salad.

> 12 ounces (340 g) pasta (fettuccine, linguine, etc.)
> 1 pound (454 g) broccoli, broken into florets
> 1 T extra virgin olive oil
> 2 large garlic cloves, finely chopped
> ¹/₄-¹/₂ t hot red pepper flakes
> 2 T pine nuts
> 4 large tomatoes, diced or 1 28-ounce (795-ml) can
>   tomatoes, chopped

Begin heating water for pasta in a large pot. When water is boiling, add the pasta, along with ¹/₂ t salt, cook until just tender and drain.

Break or cut broccoli into florets; peel and slice stems into rounds. Steam over boiling water until just tender, about 3 minutes. Set aside.

Sauté garlic, red pepper flakes and pine nuts in extra virgin olive oil in a large skillet for one minute then add tomatoes and cook medium heat 5-10 minutes. Stir in the cooked broccoli. Serve over cooked pasta.

VLF Barbara's Kale Cream Sauce over Pasta

SERVES 5

> 1 pound (454 g) pasta,cooked and drained
> 2 T whole-wheat flour
> 1 cup soy milk (1%)
> 3 T nutritional yeast
> 1/2-1 t each basil, thyme, dill, minced garlic
> salt and pepper to taste
> 1 10-ounce (284 g) package frozen kale

Heat all ingredients (except pasta) together in pan over medium heat, stirring often, until kale is done. Pour sauce over pasta and serve.

LF Pasta Primavera

SERVES 8

Vegetable mixture:
> 1 T vegetarian broth powder in water
> 1 onion, chopped
> 2 garlic cloves, minced
> 1/2 pound (227 g) mushrooms, washed and sliced
> 1 t basil
> 1/2 t oregano
> 1/4 t thyme
> 1 bell pepper, diced
> 1/4 cup fresh parsley, chopped
> 2 medium zucchini, diced
> 4 large tomatoes, finely chopped
> 1/2 t sea salt

White sauce:
> 2 T safflower oil
> 2 T flour
> 1 cup soy milk (1% or non-fat)
> 2 T nutritional yeast flakes
> 1 pound (454 g) fettuccine or other pasta

Sauté the onion in ¼ cup vegetable stock for 2 minutes then add mushrooms, garlic, and herbs and cook until mushrooms are brown. Add bell pepper, parsley, zucchini and tomatoes and cook until pepper is tender crisp, 3-5 minutes. Add salt to taste.

In a separate pan, heat the oil then stir in the flour and yeast flakes. Whisk in rice milk and cook over medium heat, stirring constantly until thickened.

Bring water to boil in a large kettle and cook pasta until tender. Place in a baking dish and sprinkle with salt and pepper. Spread white sauce over pasta then top with vegetable mixture. Bake at 350°F for 20 minutes.

LF Fettuccine with Zucchini Sauce and Fresh Tomatoes

SERVES 2

Zucchini and pasta complement each other. Add some tomatoes and basil, and this is really pasta Italiana!

> ½ pound (227 g) fettuccine or other pasta
> 2 T extra virgin olive oil
> 4 small zucchini, quartered and cut in ⅛-inch slices
> 2 T water
> ¼ t dried oregano (optional)
> 2 medium tomatoes, peeled and cubed
> 2 T fresh basil, minced or 1 t dried
> sea salt to taste
> freshly ground pepper

Prepare fettuccine according to package directions. While the pasta cooks, prepare sauce. Place oil and zucchini in a medium skillet. Sauté over medium-high heat, adding water as necessary to prevent scorching. Toss and stir zucchini for 3 minutes adding oregano as you cook. When zucchini is bright green remove from heat and set aside.

Place cooked pasta in a large bowl. Add zucchini, chopped tomatoes, fresh basil and seasonings to taste. Toss well.

LF Shepherd's Pie

SERVES 6

This is a hearty and satisfying vegetable stew with a top "crust" of fluffy mashed potatoes.

4 large potatoes, diced
$\frac{1}{2}$ cup soy milk (use 1%)
1 T margarine, or unrefined coconut butter
$\frac{1}{2}$ t salt
1 T extra virgin olive oil
2 onions, chopped
1 large bell pepper, diced
2 carrots, sliced
2 celery stalks, sliced
2 cups or $\frac{1}{2}$ pound (227 g) mushrooms, sliced
4 large tomatoes, diced
2 cups or 1 15-ounce (425-ml) can kidney beans, cooked
   and drained
$\frac{1}{2}$ t black pepper
2 T natural soy sauce
$\frac{1}{2}$ t paprika

Dice the potatoes then steam them over boiling water until tender. Mash with soy milk, margarine and salt. Set aside.

In a large skillet, sauté the onions, pepper, carrot and celery in oil for 3 minutes over medium heat. Add the mushrooms, cover the pan and cook an additional 7 minutes, stirring occasionally. Add the tomatoes, kidney beans, paprika, pepper and soy sauce, then cover and cook 10-15 minutes.

Put the vegetables into 9x13-inch baking dish and spread the mashed potatoes evenly over the top. Sprinkle with paprika. Bake at 350ºF for 25 minutes, until hot and bubbly.

ᴛᴛ Spinach Pie

Sᴇʀᴠᴇs 6

Whole-Wheat Crust:
   $1\frac{1}{4}$ cups whole-wheat pastry flour
   pinch of salt
   6 T soy or safflower margarine (non-hydrogenated)
   3-4 T ice water

Filling:
   1 t extra virgin olive oil
   1 cup onions, minced
   2 cups fresh spinach, finely chopped or 1 10-ounce
      (284g) package frozen spinach, thawed and chopped
   $\frac{1}{4}$ t grated nutmeg

1 pound (454 g) firm tofu
2 T brown rice vinegar
1 T light miso
1 T tahini
1 t Dijon-style mustard
1 garlic clove, pressed

Prepare crust. Sift flour and salt into a deep bowl. Add cold margarine, cut into small bits. Cut margarine into flour with pastry cutter or two knives until mixture resembles coarse meal. Stir in ice water with a fork and mix until dough forms into a ball. Turn out onto waxed paper and refrigerate while you prepare filling. (Pastry can actually be prepared several hours in advance and refrigerated until you are ready to use it. If prepared well in advance bring to room temperature for an hour before rolling.)

Prepare filling. Heat oil and onions in a medium skillet and sauté until translucent. Add spinach and nutmeg, and sauté one minute.

Combine tofu, vinegar, miso, tahini, mustard and garlic in a food processor or by hand and purée until creamy. Combine with spinach in a bowl and mix well by hand.

Preheat oven to 400°F. On a floured board gently roll out pie crust to fit a 9-inch pie plate. (Any cracks in the crust can be repaired once you have transferred it to the pie plate.) Crimp or flute edges. Pour filling into crust and bake for 30 minutes. Serve chilled.

TT Wayne's Tofu Chili

SERVES 8

1 pound (454 g) tofu, firm and cubed in small pieces
2 T oil
2 onions, chopped
3 green peppers, chopped
1 28-ounce (795-ml) can crushed tomatoes
1 15-ounce (425-ml) can black-eyed peas, drained
1 14-ounce (398-ml) can kidney beans, drained
1 14-ounce (398-ml) can white beans, drained
2 jalapeno peppers, minced
garlic and chili powder to taste

Sauté tofu in oil for 10 minutes. Add chopped onions and green peppers, and stir-fry 5 minutes longer. Lower heat. Add tomatoes, peas, beans, jalapeno peppers and spices. Simmer for 12 minutes. You can add some tomato paste if sauce is too thin. You can also freeze the chili to serve later.

ᴛᴛ Lentil Patties

ABOUT 12 PATTIES

> ¹/₃ cup each chopped onion and chopped bell pepper
> 1¹/₄ cups cooked lentils, mashed
> 1¹/₄ cups cooked potatoes, mashed
> ¹/₃ cup walnuts, coarse and chopped
> ¹/₄ t sage
> ¹/₄ t salt

Mix well and form into patties. Place on cookie sheet and brown in oven at 425ºF oven for 15-20 minutes. Serve plain or with gravy.

ᴠʟꜰ Black Bean Chili

SERVES 6 TO 8

This chili can be cooked on the stove or in a crockpot. Serve with brown rice or spicy bulgur pilaf and a green salad.

> 2 cups black beans
> 6 cups water
> 1 bunch cilantro, chopped
> 1 T cumin seed
> 1 T oregano
> 1 t paprika
> ¹/₂ t cayenne
> 1 large onion, chopped
> 1 T tomato juice
> 1 bell pepper, diced
> 2 garlic cloves, minced
> 1¹/₂ cups tomatoes, chopped
> ¹/₂ t salt
> ¹/₄ cup green onion, chopped

Wash beans thoroughly and remove any debris. Place in a large kettle and add the water and chopped cilantro. Cover loosely and simmer until tender, about 2 hours.

In a small dry skillet heat the herbs and toast until fragrant.

In a large skillet sauté onion in tomato juice for 3 minutes. Stir in the bell pepper, garlic and herbs and sauté until the onion is soft and golden. Add to the beans when they are tender along with the tomatoes and salt. Simmer 30 minutes or longer if time allows. The flavor improves with longer cooking.

Serve in individual bowls, topped with chopped green onion. Pass the salsa!

Crockpot method: Place washed beans in crockpot with boiling water, chopped cilantro, herbs, onion, bell pepper and garlic. Cover and cook on "high" until beans are completely tender, about 3 hours. Add chopped tomato and salt to the beans and cook at 60 minutes longer.

VLF Spicy Potatoes, Cabbage and Peas over Rice

SERVES 4

> 2 cups rice
> 4 cups water
> 5 medium potatoes, peeled, and thinly sliced
> 2 cups water
> 1/2 green cabbage
> 1 10-ounce (284 g) box of frozen peas
>   (or equivalent fresh)
> 2 t curry powder
> 1 t turmeric
> 1/2 t ginger
> 1 garlic clove, minced
> 1/8 t cayenne pepper
> salt to taste (optional)

Cook rice in 4 cups water in a covered pot over medium-high heat until done.

In a separate frying pan, add sliced potatoes to 2 cups of water and heat over medium-high heat. Shred cabbage and add to potatoes. Add peas and spices to mixture. Continue heating in covered pan, stirring occasionally, until potatoes are tender. Serve over cooked rice.

LF Mochi-Veggie Casserole

SERVES 2

Mochi is a wonderful chewy substance made out of brown rice. It is a great snack and also has the ability to melt as in this recipe. Try it!

This recipe is on the back of the sesame-garlic mochi package.

> 1 onion, chopped
> 1 t unrefined oil
> 1/3 head cabbage, chopped

1 carrot, sliced
2 T natural soy sauce
¹/₄ cup water
¹/₂ package sesame-garlic mochi

In a heavy skillet sauté onion in oil. Add cabbage, carrot, soy sauce and water. Stir. Cut mochi into one inch squares and place them on the top. Over a medium flame cover and cook 10-15 minutes until mochi melts and becomes soft and chewy.

VLF Chinese Stir-Fried Vegetables and Pineapple

SERVES 4

1 cup water
3 carrots, chopped
1 zucchini, chopped
6 ounces (170 g). snow peas
¹/₂ pound (227 g) mushrooms, chopped
2 onions, sliced
2 large tomatoes, chopped
¹/₂ pound (227 g) Mung bean sprouts
1 10-ounce (284 g) can crushed pineapple, drained
3 t natural soy sauce

Stir-fry all ingredients together over medium high-heat until carrots are tender. Serve hot with brown rice.

VLF Easy Seven-Vegetable Stew

SERVES 8 TO 10

1¹/₂ cups diced onion
1 t minced garlic
1 cup celery, diced in one inch pieces
2 T water
1 t thyme
3 T whole-wheat pastry flour
2 cups carrot rounds, in one-inch pieces
3 cups potato cubes, in one-inch pieces
1 white onion, quartered and cut in eights
3 cups water, about

1 bay leaf
dash of salt and pepper
1½ cups zucchini rounds, in one-inch pieces
1 cup frozen peas
2 cups green cabbage, chopped

Preheat oven to 325°F. Sauté diced onions, garlic and celery with 2 T water in a heavy casserole for 5 minutes stirring frequently. Add thyme and flour and stir until mixture is well coated.

Stir in carrots, potatoes and onion quarters and mix well. Add water, bring to a boil and add bay leaf and salt and pepper to taste. Cover and place in oven. Set timer for 30 minutes

Remove stew from oven. Stir in zucchini, peas and cabbage. Add a little additional water, if necessary. Replace cover and return to oven for 20 minutes. Remove from oven and adjust seasonings. Remove bay leaf.

LF Green Corn Tamale Bake

SERVES 8

The texture of this dish is wonderful.

3 cups winter squash purée
1 T extra virgin olive oil or unrefined almond oil
1 onion, diced
1 bell pepper, diced
2 garlic cloves, minced
2 cups fresh corn kernels or 2 large or small ears
2 T natural soy sauce
½ cup cornmeal

To make squash purée, either bake whole squash at 450°F until soft, about one hour, or cut squash in two-inch chunks and pressure cook 5 minutes with one cup water or steam or boil squash until done. Remove skin and seeds. Mash and measure.

Heat oil and sauté onion, pepper and garlic. Add remaining ingredients and mix well. When mixture is heated throughout spoon into corn-oiled one-quart casserole, baking dish or pie pan and bake covered for ½ hour or more.

TT My Favorite Pesto Pizza

SERVES 4

This pizza is truly delicious and so simple to prepare. Buy fresh pizza dough. This can usually be found at an Italian deli along with fresh black or green olives. For variation buy some marinated eggplant or artichokes.

Pesto sauce:
> 1¹/₂ cups basil leaves, loosely packed
> 2 garlic cloves, minced
> 1 T extra virgin olive oil
> ¹/₄ cup pine nuts, ground almonds or sunflower seeds
> 1 T fresh mild salsa

Place ingredients in a food processor and with the "S" blade blend into a paste. Roll out pizza dough. Place in a pizza pan. Spread the pesto sauce over the dough and add some or all of the following toppings depending on your taste:
> sliced mushrooms
> sliced black or green olives
> capers
> sliced onions
> sliced green, yellow or red pepper
> marinated thin strips of tofu

Do not limit yourself. Use your imagination. Kids and grownups alike love this pizza!

LF Gardin Burrito with Savory Sauce

SERVES 4

I got the idea for this dish from a restaurant in Hermosa Beach, California known as The Spot. This is a sure winner for vegetarians and non-vegetarians alike. It is also a wonderful way to use leftover beans, rice and vegetables.

> 4 whole-wheat tortillas
> 2 cups chili beans, baked beans or canned vegetarian chili or refried beans
> 2 cups brown rice, cooked
> 2 cups vegetables, steamed
> 1 cup fresh salsa

On a whole-wheat tortilla, layer the beans, rice, vegetables and salsa. Wrap it all together. Top with Savory Sauce*

Tofu Dishes

A Word about Tofu

The majority of my cooking class students either had never tasted tofu and were hesitant to do so, or they had tried cooking with it and did not want to repeat the experience! I would smile with delight when I would hear these stories because I knew that my students were in for a delightful, eyeopening surprise – they were about to fall in love with one of the most versatile and ancient food substances.

Tofu is essentially a tasteless substance made from soybeans. It picks up the flavor of whatever seasonings you add to it. It is high in protein and calcium (if calcium sulphate has been used as the coagulating agent) and an excellent transition food for those who crave a hardy substance to their meals.

A very important point about tofu is its texture and especially how to get it firm. Before you start using it with your recipe you need to remove the tofu from its packaging or from the bowl of water in which it has been kept. Slice the block of tofu wide, about ¼-inch and place it on a couple of layers of paper towels. Place another couple of layers of paper towels on the top and then perhaps a wooden chopping board or some other heavy object and allow the tofu to drain for about 1 hour. I cannot emphasize this process enough, as this has been the key for me, as well as my students, as to how much they enjoy most of their tofu dishes. Fortunately, you can find compressed tofu which has the water expressed from it, in the deli section of the natural food store. This type of firm tofu is well utilized as a meat replacement. Silken tofu has a smoother texture and is more readily suitable for sauces, puddings and cakes.

I never cease to be amazed at tofu's versatility. You will find it in the corn bread recipe, where it is used as a replacement for eggs, in the dessert section where it is used to make a delicious "cheese" cake, as a basis for yogurt, in stir-frys, lasagna, quiches and the list goes on.

If you have not done so already make sure that you get acquainted with this wonderful food.

TT Tofu Chunks or Cutlets

SERVES 4

> 2 8-ounce (227 g) cakes tofu
> 1 large onion, diced

2 garlic cloves, diced
2 T tamari
$^1/_2$ t oil
$^1/_4$ t basil
$^1/_4$ t oregano
1 cup nutritional yeast

Drain tofu well. For cutlets cut tofu into slices $^1/_4$-inch thick. For chunks, cut into 1-inch cubes. Sauté onions and garlic until golden brown. Make a mixture of tamari, oil, spices and sautéed onion and garlic. Add other favorite spices if you like.

Place tofu pieces in mixture and let marinate, then dip into nutritional yeast until thoroughly covered.

Oil a cookie sheet. Place tofu pieces on sheet and bake at 325°F for 5-7 minutes on each side, then broil until crispy. This dish can also be cooked in a frying pan with a little oil. Easy and delicious. Even quicker – leave out the onions and garlic.

Variation: Add 2 T of lemon juice to marinade mixture.

⊤⊤ Basic Quiche
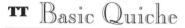

SERVES 6

14-16 ounces (398 – 454 g) tofu
$^1/_2$ cup soy milk (1%) or rice milk
1 T unrefined oil, such as olive, almond or coconut butter
1 t dijon mustard
$^1/_4$-$^1/_2$ t tumeric
2 medium onions, minced
enough oil for sautéing
salt and pepper to taste
$^1/_4$-$^1/_2$ t nutmeg, freshly grated if possible
dough for 1 whole-wheat pie crust of your choice

Cream the tofu, soy milk, oil, mustard and tumeric in a blender or food processor until absolutely smooth. Sauté the onion in oil until soft, then combine with the tofu mixture in a bowl. Season with salt, pepper and nutmeg. At this point, add various ingredients as suggested in the variations below or use as is to fill shells.

1 cup mushrooms, chopped
$^1/_2$ cup olives, chopped
$^3/_4$ cup tomatoes, chopped
1 cup mixed veggies, chopped

Roll out the crust $^1/_8$-inch thick and line a 9-inch pie pan or individual tart shells. Pre-bake the shells in a 400°F oven, 3-4 minutes for small tartlets, 10-12 minutes for a 9-inch pan. Fill with the above mixture and bake in a 350°F oven (15 minutes for individual shells or 45 minutes for a large quiche) until the top is firm and puffed up. Serve "quichettes" immediately, but wait 15 minutes before cutting a large quiche. These may also be served at room temperature.

TT Hawaiian Stir-Fry

SERVES 4 TO 6

> $^1/_4$ cup rice vinegar
> 2 T cornstarch
> $^1/_4$ cup honey
> $^1/_2$ cup vegetable stock
> saved pineapple juice
> 3 T oil
> 1 t ginger root, minced
> 1 medium onion, cut in wedges
> 1 pound (454 g) tofu, cut in $^3/_4$-inch cubes and
>   sprinkled with 3 T natural soy sauce
> 1 green pepper, cut in 1-inch triangles
> 1 sweet red pepper, cut in 1-inch triangles
> 1 15-ounce (425-ml) can unsweetened pineapple chunks,
>   drained but save the juice
> 1 5-ounce (142 g) can water chestnuts, sliced
>   and drained

Stir vinegar and cornstarch together in a small saucepan. Add honey, stock and pineapple juice. Cook and whisk over medium heat until clear and bubbly. Set aside. Heat oil in a wok or skillet, stir in ginger. Stir in the onion wedges, cook for 2 minutes, add tofu, cook for 1 minute. Add peppers and pineapple, stir. Add water chestnuts and sauce. Serve on brown rice with Chinese noodles.

TT Tofu Bourguignon

SERVES 4 TO 6

This is a lovely and tasty entrée.

> 1 pound (454 g) frozen tofu, thawed
> 1$^1/_4$ cups red wine
> 5 T mirin (Japanese seasoned rice vinegar)

5 T natural soy sauce
2-3 T miso
2 garlic cloves, minced
2 T red wine or balsamic vinegar
$^1/_2$ cup unbleached white or whole-wheat pastry flour
2 T oil
1 T extra virgin olive oil
1 medium onion, finely chopped
12 ounces (340 g) mushrooms, sliced
$^3/_4$ cup frozen peas
$^2/_3$ cup, about, rich soy cream or soy milk
1-2 t arrowroot, kuzu or cornstarch to thicken, if
  necessary

After the tofu has thawed press gently between both hands to extract as much water as possible without breaking or tearing it. Cut it into squares about $^3/_8$ x 1 x $1^1/_4$ inch. Mix the red wine, mirin, soy sauce, miso, garlic and vinegar and marinate the tofu in this mixture for at least 30 minutes (several hours if desired). Remove the tofu one piece at a time and squeeze lightly to remove some, but not all, of the marinade that it had absorbed. If you press too hard, you will end up with a tasteless piece of tofu; if you do not extract any of the marinade, the tofu may be too "winey". Measure the remaining marinade after doing this for all the pieces. You should have about $1^1/_2$ cups of marinade left. If you have too much, sprinkle some back onto the tofu; if not enough, squeeze the tofu a bit more. Flour the tofu lightly and sauté in 2 T oil on both sides until brown and crispy. Remove from the pan and set aside.

Wipe out the skillet with a paper towel and add another tablespoon of oil. Add the chopped onion, cover and sauté until tender, then add the mushrooms and cover again. Cook over low heat about five minutes until the mushroom juices being to ooze out. Add the remaining marinade and simmer for another 10 minutes. Add the green peas and cook for another two minutes. Now add the soy milk or cream and cook another minute or two to allow flavors to blend. It should thicken, but if it does not, dissolve a t or two of arrowroot or kuzu in a little more milk and add to the vegetables, stirring constantly, until the sauce has some body. Add the tofu pieces, cook another 3 minutes, then check the flavor, adjusting the seasonings and adding more soy cream, if necessary. Serve immediately over pasta, such as fettuccine, cooked al dente, or cooked rice.

TT Zesty Tofu Scramble

SERVES 4

This is a fast way to prepare tofu and can be used in many ways. Serve this for a hardy breakfast or brunch, stuff it into a pita with lettuce and tomatoes for a delicious sandwich or serve it with steamed veggies and rice for a quick dinner.

> 1 T oil
> 2 cups tofu, cubed (drain first)
> 1/2 cup red onion, diced
> 1/2 cup mushrooms, sliced
> 1/2 cup zucchini, sliced

Sauté all ingredients and season with dashes of all, some or none of the following:

basil	pepper
cilantro	natural soy sauce
dill	spike
fresh salsa	thyme

TT Korean Barbecue Tofu

SERVES 6 to 8

> 1 1/2 pounds (681 g) firm tofu
> 1/2 cup natural soy sauce
> 6 T sweetener of your choice: honey, Sucanat
>   (or turbinado sugar), Fruit sweetener, rice syrup, barley
>   malt, maple syrup or date sugar
> 2 t dry mustard
> 4 garlic cloves, minced fine
> 2 t onion powder

Cut tofu into 1/4-inch slices. Marinate at least 2 hours (overnight is best) in with remaining ingredients. Then, brown on both sides in 2 T oil. Garnish with chopped green onion, mushrooms and/or snow peas and serve with brown rice.

TT or LF Tofu Tacos

SERVES 4 TO 6

This is a fun and delicious meal for the whole family as everyone can choose the fillings for their individual taco.

½ onion, chopped or 1 T onion powder
2 garlic cloves, crushed
1 small bell pepper, diced (optional)
½ pound (227 g) firm tofu, crumbled or about 1 cup
  (fat-reduced)
1 T chili powder
1 T nutritional yeast (optional)
¼ t each cumin and oregano
1 T natural soy sauce
¼ cup tomato sauce
taco shells or corn tortillas

Garnishes:
lettuce, washed and torn
green onions, chopped
tomatoes, diced
avocado, diced
salsa or taco sauce
olives, chopped

Sauté onion, garlic and bell pepper in a non-stick pan (add a little water and soy sauce if necessary), for 2-3 minutes, then add tofu, chili powder, yeast, cumin, oregano and soy sauce. Cook 3 minutes then add tomato sauce and simmer over low heat until mixture is fairly dry.

Place a small amount of the tofu mixture in a taco and fry in 1 T oil on both sides until crisp. Garnish with lettuce, onions, tomatoes, avocado, salsa and olives.

Low-fat version: Instead of using a taco shell, warm tortillas on a dry cast-iron skillet or griddle, flipping them from side to side until they are soft and hot, then fill each with a spoonful of tofu mixture and garnish as above. Omit olives or avocado as a garnish.

TT Fresh Shiitake Stir-Fry

SERVES 4

1-inch cube fresh ginger, peeled
2 fresh garlic cloves
¼ cup mirin (Japanese rice vinegar)
3 T natural soy sauce
1 pound (454 g) firm tofu, cut in ½-inch cubes
1 T oil
½ cup scallions, sliced

1 red bell pepper, cut in triangles
3¹/₂ ounces fresh shiitake mushrooms, sliced
¹/₂ pound (227 g) snow peas, washed and stems removed

Chop ginger and garlic together in a food processor. Add the mirin and soy sauce and blend. Pour over the tofu cubes. Let this marinate while preparing vegetables. Heat oil in a wok , then, add scallions and pepper, stir-fry 1 minute. Add mushrooms and snow peas, stir-fry 1 minute. Add the tofu and marinade, stir-fry 1 minute, then cover and steam until hot. Serve over brown rice.

TT Tofu Teriyaki

SERVES 4 TO 6

1 pound (454 g) firm tofu, cut in ¹/₂-inch slabs or cubes

Teriyaki Sauce/Marinade:
1 cup natural soy sauce
¹/₂ cup brown rice vinegar
¹/₂ cup brown rice syrup or ¹/₄ cup pure maple syrup
¹/₂ cup onion, grated or minced
4 garlic cloves, crushed and minced
1 T ginger, freshly grated
1 T dry mustard powder

To prepare teriyaki sauce place ingredients in a small saucepan and heat just long enough to dissolve rice syrup.

Preheat oven to 350⁰F. (Tofu may also be barbecued or broiled.) Marinate tofu for 15 minutes. Transfer to lightly-oiled baking sheet and cook for 15-20 minutes turning once halfway through if desired.

Sauce variations: Make the following substitutions: lemon juice for vinegar; sake, mirin, or another malted grain syrup (barley malt) for part of the rice syrup; grated daikon radish or chopped green onions in place of onion; Japanese green horseradish powder (wasabi) in place of the mustard powder.

Brown Rice or Noodles with Teriyaki vegetables: Use leftover teriyaki sauce in kuzu-thickened sauces for serving over vegetables, tempeh, rice or noodles. In a small saucepan, combine ¹/₄ cup teriyaki sauce with 1 cup cool water and 1 heaping tablespoon kuzu root starch. Bring to boil and stir well until a thick sauce forms, about a minute. Makes 1¹/₄ cups. Mix sauce with 4-5 cups cooked vegetables.

LF My Tofu Scramble Mexicana

SERVES 3

I love this incredibly quick and delicious way to prepare tofu. Let your imagination go to town in thinking up ways to use this versatile dish. I always make this when I go camping.

> 1 12-ounce (340 g) package of firm tofu (fat-reduced)
> ½ t turmeric
> ½-1 cup fresh mild to hot salsa depending on
>   your preference

Mash the drained tofu and mix in the turmeric. Place on non-stick skillet over medium heat and stir. Before the tofu begins to stick, add the salsa and continue to sauté for a few minutes. That is all.

Vegetables

How many vegetables can you name? We have access to such an amazing variety , each vegetable with its own composition of vitamins, minerals, protein, water and fiber. These incredible plants with all their different colors, shapes, sizes, textures and smells are a source of life for us. Make a lot of use of them. Find ways to enjoy them. Make them at least a part of lunch and dinner. And eat them and eat them.

Eating your vegetables raw or juicing them is the most healthgiving. Steaming your vegetables so that they are still a little firm will supply you with most of the nutrients as will microwaving, although microwaving remains controversial as a method of food preparation. Baking or boiling your vegetables will yield yet less nutrients. So I do encourage you to eat your vegies raw or steamed, as much as possible.

I have enjoyed many a meal in which I simply steamed up a bunch of vegetables like cauliflower, broccoli, yams and made a tahini sauce to serve with it. It is so satisfying.

Stir-frying vegetables and serving it over brown rice is another way that I enjoy preparing vegetables.

The old saying, "Eat your vegetables, they're good for you," is simply, true.

LF Curried Spinach Salad

SERVES 6 TO 8

This salad is delicious and unusual. It is sure to impress.

> 1 bunch fresh spinach or about 1 pound (454 g)
> 1 tart green apple, diced
> 2 green onions, including green tops, finely sliced
> ¼ cup golden raisins or dried apricots, coarsely chopped
> ⅓ cup roasted Spanish peanuts
> 1 T sesame seeds, toasted
> 5 T water
> 3 T seasoned rice vinegar
> 2 t brown mustard
> 1 t natural soy sauce
> 1 t Sucanat (or turbinado sugar) or other natural
>   dry sweetener
> ½ t curry powder
> ¼ t black pepper.

Prepare the salad ingredients. Wash the spinach thoroughly making sure to remove all the sand and grit. The easiest way to do this is to submerge it in a basin of cold water and swish it around. Remove the spinach and replace the water. Repeat until no new grit shows up at the bottom of the bowl. Pat spinach dry and tear leaves into bite-sized pieces. Add apple, onion and raisins or apricots.

To roast the peanuts and sesame seeds, place them in an oven-proof pan and bake at 350ºF for 10-15 minutes. Allow to cool, then add to the salad.

For the dressing: combine water, vinegar, mustard, soy sauce, sweetener, curry powder and black pepper. Whisk together. Pour over salad and toss to mix just before serving.

VLF Lebanese Green Beans

SERVES 4

This is a particularly good recipe for mature beans, which tend to be a little tough.

> 3 T vegetable broth
> 1 large onion, sliced or diced
> 2 pounds green beans, trimmed and cut in
>   2-inch segments
> $\frac{1}{2}$ t ground cumin
> freshly ground pepper
> 1 vegetable broth cube
> 2 t sesame seeds
> lemon juice to taste

Heat the broth and add onion in a heavy skillet with a lid. Sauté, stirring frequently, until onion is soft and slightly browned. Add the green beans and water to cover. Mix well. Stir in the cumin, pepper and broth cube. Cover and cook 1 hour, stirring frequently.

When the beans are very tender and the onion has dissolved into a brown gravy sprinkle with sesame seeds and serve hot or cold, with a squeeze of lemon.

LF Mexican Style Corn

SERVES 4

> 2 10-ounce (284 g) boxes frozen corn or 8 ears
>   fresh corn, kernels cut from cob
> 2 t safflower oil

102

¼ cup red onion, diced
¼ cup green bell pepper, diced
¼ cup red bell pepper, diced
¼ to ½ t ground cumin
¼ t dried oregano

Place corn in vegetable steamer over boiling water and steam until tender, about 5-10 minutes. While corn steams heat oil and onion in a skillet. Add bell peppers and sauté 3 minutes, or until vegetables begin to soften. Add cumin and oregano, and stir-fry for 1 minute. Add steamed corn and mix well.

LF Warm Red Cabbage Salad

SERVES 4 TO 6

¼ cup walnut pieces (optional)
1 medium red onion
1 medium red cabbage
1 crisp apple
1 T extra virgin olive oil
¼ cup balsamic vinegar
1 garlic clove, finely chopped
¼ t dried marjoram or ½ t fresh marjoram
salt and fresh-ground pepper to taste
1 T fresh parsley, chopped

Place walnut pieces in a small ovenproof dish. Sprinkle with about 1 t of water then toss with salt and pepper. Bake at 350ºF for 5-7 minutes, until toasted. Cool.

Prepare vegetables: peel, quarter and slice the red onion; quarter the cabbage and remove the core; cut the cabbage into thin strips; core and dice the apple.

In a large skillet, gently heat the oil, vinegar and garlic. Do not let the garlic burn. Add the onion and cook for 30 seconds. Add the cabbage and cook, tossing gently, until it is just wilted and the color has changed from purple to bright pink.

Remove the pan from heat and season salad with marjoram, salt and freshly ground pepper. Add parsley, apple and walnuts and toss gently to mix.

VLF Corn Relish

SERVES 9 OR 3¹/₄ CUPS

> 2 cups fresh corn kernels, yellow or part white
> ¹/₂ cup celery
> ¹/₂ cup onion
> ¹/₂ cup apple cider vinegar
> ¹/₂ cup apple juice
> 1¹/₂ t mustard powder
> 1 t sea salt
> ¹/₂ t celery seed
> ¹/₂ cup green bell pepper
> ¹/₂ cup red bell pepper

Dice vegetables to size of corn. Place all ingredients, except bell peppers, in a 2-quart pot. Bring to boil, then slow boil covered for 5 minutes, stirring occasionally, Add bell peppers in last 2 minutes of cooking to preserve color. Allow to cool, then drain just before serving.

May be preserved by canning or refrigerate.

LF Vegetables with Italian Herb Paste Pesto

SERVES 6 TO 8

> Vegetables:
> > 1 medium carrot, cut in 1¹/₂-inch pieces across, then in
> > ¹/₄-inch slices length-wise
> > 1 medium red onion, halved from top to bottom, then
> > cut in ¹/₄-inch slices or crescents
> > 1¹/₂ cups cauliflower, separated into bite-size florets,
> > stems and core cut in ¹/₄-inch slices
> > 1¹/₂ cups broccoli, tops separated into bite-size florets,
> > edible portion of stems cut like carrots,
> > hard skin discarded
> > 1 cup green beans, (or peas with edible pods) ends
> > discarded, beans cut in thirds, about ¹/₄ pound
> > ¹/₂ cup Italian Herb paste (Pesto)

> Italian Herb Paste (Pesto): makes 1-1¹/₄ cups
> > 2 cups fresh basil, about 1 bunch, stems and any

discolored leaves discarded, gently packed
2 large garlic cloves, chopped
$^1/_2$ cups walnuts or pine nuts, lightly toasted
$^1/_4$ cup water
1 t extra virgin olive oil
1 t sea salt or 2 T natural soy sauce, or half of each

To prepare pesto, blend ingredients until smooth.

To prepare vegetables, quick-boil (about 5 minutes) or steam (about 8-15 minutes) until done. Vegetables may be cooked together except green beans which may take longer. Gently mix vegetables to distribute colors evenly. Spoon a dollop of pesto atop each serving or mix into vegetables in serving bowl, reserving a few undressed vegetables to place on top for color clarity.

VLF Vegetables with Dill

SERVES 2 TO 4

1 large broccoli stalk, chopped
$^1/_2$ head cauliflower, chopped
2 red potatoes (about 1$^1/_2$ cups), cubed
2 T dill, fresh and minced
1 T chives, fresh and minced
1 T lemon juice
1 T Bragg Liquid Aminos or natural soy sauce
2 T water from steaming

Steam veggies. Blend dill, chives, lemon juice, liquid aminos and seasoned water. Pour over vegetables and toss.

LF Mushroom Ratatouille

SERVES 3

Hot or cold, this is a great topping for grains, potatoes and pasta

1 T extra virgin olive oil
1 t dried thyme
1 t dried oregano
$^1/_2$ cup red onion, finely chopped
1 pound (454 g) mushrooms, ends trimmed and caps
thinly sliced
1 cup or 1 large fresh or canned tomato, peeled
and chopped

ground rock salt
freshly ground black pepper

Heat the oil, spices and onion in a skillet. Add mushrooms and sauté until natural juices form. Add chopped tomatoes and salt and pepper to taste.

VLF Broccoli with Mustard Sauce

SERVES 4 TO 6

1 bunch broccoli
2 T Dijon mustard
2 T seasoned rice vinegar
2 T rice syrup or 1 T mild honey

Break the broccoli into bite-sized florets. Peel the stems and slice them into 1/4-inch thick rounds. Steam until just tender, about 3 minutes.

While the broccoli is steaming, combine the remaining ingredients in a serving bowl. Add the steamed broccoli and toss to mix.

LF Sesame Carrots with Dill Weed

SERVES 2 TO 4

6 carrots, peeled and thinly sliced
2 cups water
1 t dill weed
2 t sesame oil
2 t sesame seeds (optional)

Heat carrots in water for approximately 10 minutes over a medium-high heat in a large uncovered frying pan, until most of the water evaporates. Carrots will be slightly tender. Reduce heat to low. Add dill weed, sesame oil and sesame seeds if desired. Heat 2 minutes longer and serve.

VLF Creamed Spinach

SERVES 4

1 10-ounce (284 g) box frozen spinach, chopped
1/2 cup water
1 cup soy milk (1% or non-fat)
1/4 t nutmeg
1 garlic clove, minced
1 t natural soy sauce
1 T cornstarch, mix with water then add

Cook spinach in water over medium heat for 15 minutes. Add remaining ingredients and simmer over medium-low heat for 3 minutes longer, stirring often.

VLF Sautéed Spinach with Water Chestnuts

SERVES 2

> 1 10-ounce (284 g) bag fresh spinach, washed and chopped
> 1 T vegetable broth
> 1/3 cup water
> 2 garlic cloves, minced
> 1/2 t cumin
> 1/8 t cayenne pepper
> 1 T lemon juice
> 4 ounces (114 g) water chestnuts, thinly sliced

Sauté all ingredients over medium-high heat for 5 minutes.

VLF Zucchini Pancakes

SERVES 4

> 1 medium zucchini
> 1 small onion
> 1/2 cup water
> 1 cup whole-wheat pastry flour
> 1 garlic clove
> 1 T parsley flakes
> 1 t tamari or natural soy sauce

Blend zucchini, onion and water in a food processor. Pour into a bowl and add flour, garlic, parsley and soy sauce. Form ten small pancakes and fry in an oiled pan over medium heat. Brown both sides. A light coating of an unrefined oil should do the trick for frying.

VLF Steamed Squash

> 2 yellow squash, thinly sliced
> 2 zucchini, thinly sliced
> 1 T natural soy sauce or tamari
> 1 t nutritional yeast

1 t dill weed

Steam yellow squash and zucchini for 10-15 minutes (depending on how tender you prefer your vegetables). Remove squash and place in a dish. Sprinkle with soy sauce or tamari, nutritional yeast and dill weed.

VLF Herbed Cabbage Medley

SERVES 3

> 1 medium onion, thinly sliced
> ½ small head cabbage, shredded or about three cups
> 3 medium carrots, shredded or about 1½ cups
> ½ t salt
> ½-1 t oregano

Cook onion in a small amount of water for 5 minutes. Add the cabbage and carrots and salt. Cover, cook over medium heat for 6-8 minutes more. Stir in crushed oregano.

VLF Broccoli Italiano

SERVES 4

> 1 bunch broccoli
> 1 garlic clove
> ½ cup water
> 1 T vegetarian broth powder
> 1 2-ounce (57-ml) jar pimentos
> salt to taste

Remove the leaves from the broccoli and cut off the lower part of the stalk. Combine the vegetable broth powder with the water. Cut broccoli into florets, rinse and drain. Sauté the garlic and broccoli for five minutes using ¼ cup of the broth mixture. Discard the garlic. Add the rest of the broth. Salt to taste. Cover and cook over low heat for 10-15 minutes, or until broccoli is tender, adding a little more water if the skillet dries out. Sprinkle with pimentos and serve.

Grains and Potatoes

I love grains and potatoes. They really provide the body with needed fuel and they taste so good! When I used to go out for breakfast and order eggs and hashbrowns I always loved the potatoes more.

I have included many recipes for potatoes that are healthy. All general cookbooks have potato recipes, but most are laden with fat and salt. These recipes are low in fat and delicious.

When you are using grains make sure to wash them first. I place my grains in a strainer and run water over them.

There are so many grains to choose from: brown rice, oats, millet, barley, buckwheat, cracked wheat, corn, rye, quinoa, spelt, teff, amaranth and more, each with its own character and flavor and each with its own cooking requirements.

Always cook more than you need. You will find wonderful uses for the extra such as grain salads, puddings, adding to soups, in casseroles, in veggie-burgers and patties and in sandwich wraps. To soften it after storage just place it on a steamer and steam for a few minutes.

Note: for more information please refer to grain cooking chart on page 26.

LF Potato Boats

SERVES 2 TO 3

> 3 large potatoes, cleaned
> 2 cups rice milk
> seasonings: garlic, oregano, paprika, natural soy sauce
>   or your other favorite herbs

Bake potatoes and allow to cool, spoon out insides onto large platter leaving skins intact. Mash with fork and add rice milk until right consistency. Season as desired. Spoon mixture into potato shells and place chopped pimento or onion on top. Bake at 350ºF for 20 minutes.

TT Potato Latkes

SERVES 2

Serve with applesauce or ketchup.

> ½ cup firm tofu
> ¾ cup soy milk (non-fat)
> 3 T flour

1 T onion powder
2 small potatoes
¹/₄ onion

Purée tofu in blender, add soy milk. Shred or grate potatoes and onion in food processor, squeeze excess liquid from vegetables and blot dry. Put tofu and shredded vegetables in bowl, stir together with flour and onion powder. Pour mix onto hot oiled griddle and flip when brown.

LF Mashed Potatoes and Gravy

SERVES 6

4 large potatoes, peeled and diced
1¹/₂ cups water
¹/₂ t salt
¹/₂ cup soy milk (1% or non-fat) or rice milk
¹/₂ cup onion,chopped
1 cup mushrooms,sliced
2 T flour
2 t natural soy sauce
¹/₄ t black pepper

Place potatoes in kettle with water and ¹/₄ t salt. Cover and simmer until potatoes are tender, about 10 minutes. Drain and reserve liquid. Mash the potatoes then add remaining salt and soy milk. Cover and set aside.

In a large skillet sauté onions and mushrooms until onions are soft and transparent. Stir in flour; the mixture will be quite dry. Whisk in cooking liquid from potatoes then add soy sauce and pepper. Cook over medium-low heat until thickened.

Serve over the mashed potatoes.

VLF Simple Fat~Free Potato Puffs

Use organic red- or yellow-skinned potatoes. Wash. Slice into ¹/₄-inch rounds. Preheat oven or toaster oven to 375⁰F. Place slices on racks. Bake until puffed up, approximately 15 minutes. Serve plain or with healthy ketchup or sprinkle with garlic or a little rice vinegar.

This recipe was contributed by Marilyn Barnes.

LF Mediterranean Oven Fries

From my friend Jia Patton who created most of the recipes for John Robbins' book, *May All Be Fed*, comes this non-fat method for potato "fries".

4-6 small new potatoes or 2 large baking potatoes, cut in ¼-inch slices
2 T tamari
2 T fresh basil, finely chopped (2 t dried basil)
1 T fresh oregano, finely chopped (1 t dried oregano)
1 T fresh lemon juice
1 garlic clove, pressed or minced
pinch of cayenne

Toss all ingredients and bake on the middle rack at 400ºF. (Use a non-stick or a lightly oiled baking sheet.) Bake for 20 minutes, turn potatoes at 10 minutes.

LF Easy Oven-Baked Hash Browns

SERVES 3 TO 4

6 large red-skinned potatoes, steamed, peeled and thinly sliced
1 small onion, diced
2 large garlic cloves, minced
1 T unrefined oil
ground rock salt and freshly ground pepper to taste
paprika to taste
1 T minced parsley

Preheat oven to 450ºF. Place potatoes in lightly oiled baking dish. Add onion, garlic, oil and salt and pepper. Toss well. Dust lightly with paprika and parsley. Bake 15 minutes. Turn with a spatula. Lower heat to 350ºF and bake 30 minutes to an hour longer. Potatoes can remain in warm (300ºF) oven for up to two hours or until you are ready to eat.

VLF Couscous

MAKES 3 CUPS

This grain, a type of wheat, is very easy and quick to prepare.

1½ cups boiling water
½ t salt
1 cup couscous

Place water and salt into a small saucepan and bring to a boil. Stir in the couscous, remove from heat and cover the pan. Let stand 10-15 minutes, then fluff with a fork and serve.

LF Bulgur Wheat Salad (Tabouli)

MAKES 3 CUPS

This is a real favorite of mine and I usually make it from scratch. However buying it in a package has given me very satisfactory results. Tabouli teams up beautifully with hummus in whole-wheat pita pockets with sprouts and tomatoes.

> 1 cup bulgur wheat
> 1/2 cup boiling water
> 1/2 t sea salt
> 1 cup cucumber, diced small
> 1/2 cup parsley, finely sliced
> 1/2 cup green onion, finely sliced
> lettuce leaves for serving (optional)
> 2 tomatoes, chopped

Lemon-Garlic Mint Dressing: makes 6-7 T
> 1/4-1/3 cup lemon juice, to taste (start with less)
> 1/2 T extra virgin olive oil
> 1 garlic clove, minced
> 1 T fresh mint leaves, minced

Place bulgur and salt in a saucepan or bowl, then add boiling water. Cover and let stand 20 minutes, until all water is absorbed. Transfer to a large bowl by fluffing with a fork, and allow to cool.

To prepare dressing, mix ingredients well. Gently mix bulgur with vegetables and dressing. Serve as is or on individual lettuce leaves.

To increase volume (as for 10 times this recipe) multiply ingredients proportionately, except water which should be measured to 1 inch above bulgur.

LF Spicy Bulgur Pilaf

SERVES 4 TO 6

Serve with chili or refried beans and a green salad.

> 1 T extra virgin olive oil
> 1 medium onion, chopped
> 2 cloves garlic, crushed
> 1 cup bulgur wheat
> 2 t chili powder
> 3/4 t ground cumin

$^1/_8$ t celery seed
$^1/_2$ red bell pepper, finely diced
$^1/_2$ t salt
1$^1/_2$ cups boiling water or vegetable stock

Heat oil in a large skillet, then add onion, garlic and bulgur and cook 2-3 minutes, stirring frequently. Stir in the chili powder, cumin, celery seed, and continue cooking 3-5 minutes.

Add the bell pepper and salt, then pour in the boiling water (or stock). Bring to a boil then reduce to a simmer. Cover and cook, without stirring, until all liquid is absorbed, about 20 minutes.

Oven method: Prepare all ingredients as above, up to the addition of boiling water or stock. Preheat oven to 350°F. Place bulgur mixture into an ovenproof dish, pour in boiling liquid, cover with foil and bake in preheated oven for 30 minutes, until all liquid is absorbed.

VLF Chinese Fried Bulgur

SERVES 6

Another bulgur recipe as this grain is so easy to prepare and so versatile. Perfect with any vegetable stir-fry.

1 cup bulgur
$^1/_4$ t salt
1$^3/_4$ cups boiling water
1 t fresh minced ginger
$^1/_2$ cup finely sliced green onions, including tops
$^1/_4$ cup vegetarian broth powder
1 t sesame oil
$^1/_2$ cup sliced water chestnuts
1$^1/_2$ T natural soy sauce
$^1/_8$ t black pepper

Place bulgur and salt in a saucepan or bowl then add boiling water. Cover and let stand 20 minutes until all water is absorbed.

In large skillet, sauté ginger and onion in broth for one minute. Add sesame oil, water chestnuts, soaked bulgur, soy sauce and pepper and continue cooking until everything is hot.

VLF Perfect Spanish Rice

SERVES 6

> ¼ cup water
> ½ cup onion, chopped
> ½ t ground coriander
> ¼ (scant) t ground cumin
> 1 T dehydrated vegetables (optional)
> 2 t powdered vegetable broth, 1 vegetable bouillon cube, or 2 t yellow miso (light)
> 2 cups white or brown basmati rice, washed and drained
> 4 cups water
> ¾ t salt-free seasoning
> 1 medium tomato
> 1½ cups frozen petite peas
> freshly ground pepper

Heat water in a medium saucepan with a lid. Add onion and sauté until translucent over medium-low heat. Add the coriander and cumin and sauté, stirring constantly, for 1 minute. Add dehydrated vegetables, broth powder, and rice to saucepan. Mix thoroughly.

Add water and ½ t salt-free seasoning then bring to a boil, stirring frequently. Cover and reduce heat to low. Simmer 20 minutes for white basmati, 35 minutes for brown basmati. Plunge tomato into boiling water for 30 seconds or until skin loosens. Peel and chop or purée with hand blender or in food processor. When rice is ready stir in peas and tomato. Add remaining salt-free seasoning and pepper to taste. Mix thoroughly but gently, cover and cook over low heat an additional 3 minutes to cook peas.

LF Tofu Corn Bread

SERVES 8

This cornbread goes very nicely with stews and bean chilis.

> 1 cup cornmeal
> 1 cup flour (unbleached or whole wheat pastry)
> 2 T turbinado sugar or other sweetener
> ¾ t salt
> 1 t baking powder
> ½ t baking soda
> ¼ pound tofu or ½ cup (fat-reduced)
> 1½ cups water
> 1½ T rice vinegar
> 2 T oil

Preheat oven to 425°F.

Mix dry ingredients in a large bowl. Combine liquid ingredients in blender and blend until smooth. Pour liquid ingredients into flour mixture and stir until just blended.

Spread evenly in a greased and floured 9x9-inch baking dish, and bake at 425°F for 25-30 minutes. Serve hot.

Dressings and Toppings

A good salad dressing can make a salad eater out of almost everyone. I have included many in this collection. Try them and find the ones you really like and enjoy them.

Sweet toppings can be used in so many ways: to dress up a plain baked apple, to add to grains for an instant dessert, on pancakes, waffles, or french toast.

TT Herbed Olive Oil Dressing

MAKES ¾ CUP

> ⅓ cup extra virgin olive oil
> 3 T wine vinegar
> 2 T parsley, chopped
> ¼ t kelp powder
> ¼ t pepper
> enough water to make one cup

Mix together thoroughly.

TT Tahini Dressing or Dip

MAKES 2 CUPS

This is my all-time favorite and I use it in salads, on steamed vegetables and grains. Sesame seeds are high in calcium and protein.

> 1 cup sesame tahini
> 2 T lemon juice
> ⅔ cup water
> 1 T minced onion
> 1 garlic clove, minced
> 2 T natural soy sauce or tamari
> 2 T sweetener

Mix together thoroughly.
For a dip reduce water to ½ cup.

VLF Quick Salsa

SERVES 8

> 1 29-ounce (795-ml) can tomatoes, drained
> 2 ripe tomatoes

1 green pepper
4 scallions
1 small jalapeno pepper, finely chopped
1 large fresh garlic clove, minced
juice of one fresh lime
salt to taste (optional)

Pulse all the ingredients together in a food processor. Be sure to pulse briefly. Serve with chips.

VLF Ketchup

MAKES ABOUT 12 OUNCES

1 12-ounce (340-ml) can tomato paste
2 T date sugar or date butter
½ t salt.
2 T lemon juice
¼ t onion powder
1 small garlic clove, minced

Just mix together. Quick, easy and very tasty.

TT Garlic-Herb Dressing for a Crowd

SERVES 20

1½ cups extra virgin olive oil
½ cup fresh lemon juice
10 medium garlic cloves
2 t paprika
2 t dried basil
2 t dried mint
2 t dried thyme
1 t dried oregano
1 t dried chervil
¼ cup seasoned salt

Measure half the ingredients into a blender and blend until smooth and creamy, taking care that garlic breaks down entirely. (You do not want people to receive a hunk of garlic in their mouth while enjoying your salad.) Measure the second half of the ingredients into the blender and repeat.

Variations: add 4 T of Dijon-style mustard for tangier dressing (reduce the amount of seasoned salt by ¼ or add 4 T tahini and ½ cup water.

117

TT Thousand Island Dressing

MAKES 1³/₄ CUPS

> ¹/₂ pound (227 g) tofu, mashed
> ¹/₂ cup ketchup
> ¹/₂ t onion powder
> ¹/₄ t salt
> 1 small garlic clove, minced
> 3 T sweet pickle relish
> 3 T stuffed green olives, minced
> 1 T parsley, finely chopped

Combine tofu, ketchup, onion powder, salt and garlic in a blender and blend until smooth and creamy. Fold in remaining ingredients.

LF Dill Salad Dressing

MAKES 1¹/₄ CUPS

> ¹/₂ pound (227 g) tofu, mashed (fat-reduced)
> 1 T wine vinegar
> ¹/₂ t dill weed
> ¹/₂ t salt
> ¹/₈ t black pepper

Combine in a blender. Blend until smooth and creamy.

LF Green Goddess Dressing

MAKES 1³/₄ CUPS

> ¹/₂ pound (227 g) tofu, mashed (fat-reduced)
> ¹/₂ T dry chives
> ¹/₄ cup fresh parsley
> 2 T wine vinegar
> 1 t onion powder
> ¹/₂ t salt
> ¹/₂ garlic clove, minced
> ¹/₈ t black pepper

Combine in blender. Blend until smooth and creamy.

LF Creamy Italian Dressing

MAKES 1¹/₄ CUPS

> ¹/₂ pound (227 g) tofu (fat-reduced)

1 T wine vinegar
1 t salt
$^1/_8$ t freshly ground black pepper
4 garlic cloves, minced
2 T sweet pickle relish (optional)
$^1/_4$ t oregano
$^1/_8$ t red pepper flakes

Combine tofu, vinegar, salt and pepper in a blender. Blend until smooth and creamy. Fold in remaining ingredients.

LF Russian Dressing

MAKES 1$^1/_2$ CUPS

$^1/_2$ pound (227 g) soft tofu (fat-reduced)
$^1/_3$ cup ketchup
2 T wine vinegar
1 T prepared mustard
1 t onion powder
$^1/_2$ t salt

Combine in blender. Blend until smooth and creamy.

VLF Basic Free Dressing

MAKES 1 CUP

$^1/_2$ cup apple cider vinegar or wine vinegar
$^1/_2$ cup water
$^1/_2$ t dry mustard
$^1/_2$ t pepper
1 t celery seed
1 t dill seed

Mix together thoroughly.

VLF Fat-Free Salad Dressing

MAKES $^1/_2$ CUP

$^1/_2$ cup seasoned rice vinegar
1-2 t Dijon-style mustard
1 garlic clove, pressed

Whisk all ingredients together. Use as a dressing on green salads and steamed vegetables.

VLF Light Lemon-Rice Vinegar Dressing

MAKES 2 T

    1 T lemon juice
    1 T brown rice vinegar

Mix ingredients.

VLF 2-Taste Dressing

MAKES 2 T

    2 T brown rice vinegar or lemon juice
    2 T natural soy sauce

Mix ingredients.

TT Tomato Herb Dressing

MAKES $^3/_4$ CUP

    1 large ripe tomato
    1 T lemon juice
    $^1/_4$ cup extra virgin olive oil
    $^1/_2$ t dried tarragon or 1$^1/_2$ t fresh
    1 T fresh basil or 1 t dried
    dash of Worcestershire sauce
    dash of cayenne
    salt-free seasoning to taste (optional)

Mix ingredients.

TT Lemon-Poppy Seed Dressing

SERVES 3 TO 4

    1$^1/_2$ T poppy seeds
    2$^1/_2$ T lemon juice
    1 t honey or Fruit Source
    2 T dairy-free mayonnaise
    $^1/_2$ t dry mustard
    1$^1/_2$ T unrefined sunflower oil

Mix ingredients.

TT Tofu Mayonnaise

MAKES ABOUT 2 CUPS

$^1\!/_2$ cup unrefined safflower oil
1 cup apple cider vinegar
1$^1\!/_2$ cakes soft tofu (8 ounces each)
$^1\!/_3$ cup fructose
1$^1\!/_2$ T lemon juice
1 T sea salt

Mix ingredients.

Gravies and Sauces

All I can say about this section is to build your repertoire. The more gravies and sauces that you know, the more ordinary meals you can turn into delightful dining experiences. Plain brown rice can suddenly become a sweet dessert, or an East Indian, Chinese, Italian, Mexican delight, to name a few. They are truly magical because of their transformational powers.

Be flexible with recipes, season to your taste. There are a variety of thickeners: cornstarch, arrowroot powder and kuzu. You can use these interchangeably. Always dissolve the powder in a little water first before adding to the main ingredients.

LF Country Gravy

MAKES 12 SERVINGS OR 1¹/₂ CUPS

> 2 T sunflower oil (or other kind)
> ¹/₃ cup whole-wheat pastry flour
> 2 cups cool water
> 1 T natural soy sauce
> 1 t sea salt
> 1 T fresh sage, minced, or 1¹/₂ t dried, crushed
> 2 T parsley, minced

To prepare Country Gravy, in a skillet or saucepan heat oil, add flour, and stir until oil is completely absorbed. Set pan aside to cool, about 15 minutes. Mix remaining ingredients except parsley and gradually add liquid to flour, stirring with a wire whisk to avoid lumping. (Gravy should be no more than 1 inch deep in pan in order for it to cook in this brief amount of time.) When all liquid is added, bring mixture to a boil, stirring occasionally. Lower heat to simmer uncovered until desired consistency is reached, about 10-15 minutes. Stir in parsley in last 2 minutes of cooking. (For larger amounts, increase ingredients proportionately, but allow more time for cooking, about ¹/₂ hour for 4X recipe.)

VLF Brown or Chicken-Like Gravy

ABOUT 4 CUPS

> 1 onion, diced
> ¹/₄ cup water and 3 T whole-wheat flour
> 3 cups potato or green bean water

1 T Vegix, Marmite or Vegemite, soy sauce or "Chicken"

Style Seasoning* to taste.

Blend and bring to a boil..

Variation: For creamy gravy add ½ cup cashews to the mixture and blend, using a little "Chicken" Style Seasoning*.

LF Basic Vegetarian Gravy

1 large onion
1 T extra virgin olive oil
2 T natural soy sauce
4 T whole-wheat flour
4 cups water or soup stock
1 vegetable bouillon cube or
1 T vegetable broth powder
1 T nutritional yeast flakes or powder
2 T cashews or almonds, ground or roasted
   sunflower seeds
⅛ t black pepper
vegetable salt to season

Sauté onions in oil until golden brown. Add soy sauce and simmer for about one more minute on low heat. Dissolve whole-wheat flour in two cups of cold water. Bring remaining water to a boil and add flour mixture stirring constantly. Let simmer on low heat while adding bouillon cube or powder, yeast flakes, sautéd onions and ground nuts. Blend well to make a smooth gravy. Add spices and season to taste using more powdered vegetable broth or sea salt if desired.

Variations:

Add three cloves of garlic to make a garlic gravy.

For mushroom gravy, sauté two cups of sliced mushrooms in one T olive oil and one T soy sauce for about five to ten minutes. Either add the sliced mushrooms to gravy or, for creamy mushroom gravy, blend them before adding to the gravy.

For horseradish gravy, add one to two T freshly ground horseradish before serving.

Substitutes:

Whole-wheat flour can be substituted with rice, spelt or barley flour or one large potato, finely grated. (Simmer the gravy a bit longer to make sure potato is cooked.)

Gravy can be thickened with ½ cup cooked millet or quinoa instead of flour.

* Recipe in Recipe Collection

VLF Fat-Free Gravy

MAKES 1¼ CUPS

> 1 cup water or stock
> 2 T miso
> 2 T natural soy sauce
> ½ t celery seeds
> 2-3 T nutritional yeast
> freshly ground pepper to taste
> 3 T cornstarch mixed with enough water to dissolve

Combine all ingredients except the cornstarch mixture and bring to a simmer for 5 minutes. Add the cornstarch mixture a little at a time stirring constantly until thickened.

VLF Pasta with Carrot-Ginger Sauce

SERVES 6

> 1½ to 2 cups water
> 1 pound (454 g) carrots, cut in pieces
> 1 medium onion, chopped
> 2 T Bragg Liquid Aminos (to taste)
> 2 T grated ginger (to taste)
> 3 or 4 garlic cloves, chopped
> 1 tomato, diced
> 2 to 3 cups diced vegetables (summer squash, broccoli)

Heat water. Add carrots, onion and liquid aminos. Cover and simmer for 12-15 minutes. Add ginger and garlic. Cover and simmer for 5-10 minutes. Remove from heat. Place vegetables and liquid in blender. Blend until smooth. Return to pot on medium heat. Add diced vegetables. Cook for 5-10 minutes. Serve over favorite pasta, or rice.

LF Savory Sauce

SERVES 4 TO 6

This sauce is definitely one of my favorites as it is extremely versatile and easy to prepare. I first tasted a version of it at The Spot, a wonderful little restaurant in Hermosa Beach, California. I have reduced some of the fat from the original recipe. Serve this sauce over pasta, grains, steamed veggies, burritos - use your imagination!

> 12 ounces firm tofu (fat-reduced)
> ¾ cup water

¼ cup natural soy sauce or tamari
4 T nutritional yeast flakes
1-2 garlic cloves, minced
¼ cup unrefined almond oil
1 T lemon juice
½ t basil
½ t salt
½ t kelp

Place all ingredients in a blender and blend until smooth and creamy. Heat and serve. This sauce can also be frozen for later use.

LF Golden Sauce

SERVES 4

¾ cup cooked potato
1 medium carrot, cooked
1⅓ cups water
2 T cashews
¾ t salt
1 T lemon juice

Blend in blender until smooth. Heat and serve over vegetables such as cauliflower, broccoli, eggplant and baked potatoes.

LF Chickpea Sauce

SERVES 4

1 19-ounce can chickpeas (garbanzo beans), drained (or 2 cups cooked chickpeas)
1 15-ounce (425-ml) can tomato sauce
1 6-ounce (170-ml) can tomato paste
1 t onion powder
1 T basil
pinch of black pepper
salt to taste

Simmer ingredients for 5 minutes over low heat, stirring occasionally. When hot pour over cooked spinach pasta or other type of pasta.

VLF Ginger Sauce

MAKES 2¼ CUPS

2 t fresh ginger, peeled and grated
2 cups water

125

¼ cup natural soy sauce
¼ cup kuzu root starch

Place ingredients in small saucepan. Stir to dissolve kuzu. Bring to boil, stirring gently, until a sauce thickens (several minutes).

LF Fresh Tomato-Basil Sauce

SERVES 4

This is a fabulous sauce when organic ripe tomatoes are in season. Serve with any type of pasta.

8 cups or about 5 pounds very ripe tomatoes, chopped
and peeled
1 T extra virgin olive oil
1 cups onions, chopped
2 garlic cloves, minced
3 T fresh basil leaves, finely chopped or 1 T dried basil
1 T sugar, honey or other sweetener
salt and pepper to taste
1 6-ounce (170-ml) can tomato paste

Place chopped tomatoes in a colander or strainer for 30 minutes to drain. Press down with a spoon several times to squeeze out excess liquid.

In a medium saucepan heat oil over medium heat. Add onions and garlic and cook until onions are tender, 5-10 minutes.

Add tomatoes, basil, sweetener, salt and pepper to saucepan and bring to a boil. Reduce heat to low and simmer, uncovered, 1 hour. Stir in tomato paste and continue to cook 10 more minutes.

LF Vegetarian Spaghetti Sauce

SERVES 4 TO 6

I love this sauce! It freezes very well, so make lots.

3 garlic cloves, pressed
1 medium onion, chopped
1 T extra virgin olive oil
1 28-ounce (795-ml) can whole tomatoes
2 medium zucchini, diced
1 6-ounce (170-ml) can tomato paste
2 T basil
1 t oregano

1 t salt and pepper
1 t sweetener

Sauté garlic and onion in oil. Add the whole tomatoes and zucchini. Add the paste and the spices. Let simmer before determining how many paste cans of water to add. Simmer 2-3 hours. Add more garlic to taste.

Variations: The wonderful thing about vegetarian spaghetti sauce is how adaptable it is. According to your mood, add:

grated carrots
sunflower seeds, for texture
tofu, crumbled and fried
green pepper or broccoli
$\frac{1}{4}$ cup red wine

VLF Lemon Sauce

MAKES 1 CUP

1 cup unsweetened pineapple juice
1 T lemon juice
1 t vanilla
2 T cornstarch

Mix ingredients in saucepan and cook over medium heat until thick; stirring as necessary to keep smooth. Pour over baked apple dish. Serve hot or cold.

VLF Strawberry Sauce

MAKES 2$\frac{1}{2}$ CUPS

1 T arrowroot or cornstarch
1 cup pineapple juice
1$\frac{1}{2}$ cups strawberries

Mix starch with some of the pineapple juice. Heat rest of pineapple juice to boiling point than add the starch mixture. Stir until thick. Add strawberries and serve.

VLF Orange Date Sauce

MAKES 2$\frac{1}{2}$ CUPS

2 cups dates
2 cups water
$\frac{1}{2}$ cup orange juice

Cook dates in water until soft. Blend date mixture with 1 cup orange juice. Serve over waffles, French toast, etc.

Desserts

You can see from the sheer volume of recipes in this section that I am a dessert fan. Not surprising, given the fact that my father was a baker.

Making desserts without any dairy products or eggs in them is a little challenging on your own. These recipes are simple to prepare and delicious to eat. I made sure to test all of these!

Some important baking tips:

> To replace eggs: in baking, use egg replacer, which you will find in the natural food stores, or half a ripe banana or 1/4 cup of tofu.

> To replace milk: in baking, use almond, cashew or sunflower milk, or soy milk.

> To replace white sugar: use maple syrup, barley malt, rice syrup or date sugar. These items can be found in the natural food store.

> To replace butter: in baking, use nut butters instead – almond, cashew, hazelnut, peanut.

Try adapting some of your old favorites to the more healthful way of eating desserts. Those of you with a sweet tooth will not be wanting. I know.

LF Oatmeal-Almond Pie Crust

MAKES 2 CRUSTS

> 1½ cup oatmeal, ground to flour
> ¾ cup almonds, ground
> ¼ cup sesame seeds, ground
> ¼ t salt
> ⅓-½ cup water for soft dough

Mix first four ingredients and then add water. Mix lightly and dust with oatmeal flour. Roll out 2 crusts and put in pie pans. Bake at 375⁰F degrees for 10-15 minutes, watching carefully. It should be slightly brown. Cool before adding the cooled filling.

VLF Fat-Free Pie Crust

MAKES 1 CRUST

This crust is slightly sweet and chewy. I use it regularly as a substitute for crumb crusts, and often find it appropriate in place of a regular pastry crust. In addition to being fat-free, it is blessedly easy to prepare.

2 cups Grape-Nuts cereal
$\frac{1}{2}$ cup apple juice concentrate (undiluted)

Preheat oven at 350ºF. Mix the Grape-Nuts and apple juice concentrate. Pat into a pie pan and bake at 350ºF for 10 minutes. Cool and fill as directed.

VLF American Berry Pie

SERVES 10

The bright red and blue of the berries make this a very festive summer desert that brings "oohs" and "aahs!"

Filling:
2 pints strawberries
$\frac{1}{2}$ t sea salt
$\frac{1}{2}$ cup rice syrup
$\frac{1}{2}$ cup agar sea vegetable flakes
1 pint blueberries

Basic Single Crust Pie Dough:
$1\frac{1}{2}$ cups whole-wheat pastry flour
$\frac{1}{2}$ cup water
$1\frac{1}{2}$ T unrefined coconut butter or almond oil
$\frac{1}{4}$ t sea salt

To prepare filling, rinse strawberries by placing in a bowl of cool water, swishing them quickly and removing them. Pinch off stems after rinsing or some of the flavorful juice will be lost in the water. Cut only very large berries in half. Leave others whole.

Place strawberries in saucepan and sprinkle with salt. Pour rice syrup over and sprinkle agar flakes over all. Cover pan and bring to boil then simmer until agar is completely dissolved, around 15 minutes. Strawberries are so full of liquid (about $\frac{1}{2}$ cup comes out) that no added liquid is necessary as long as you keep the flame at medium-low. Stir several times. Add blueberries in last five minutes of cooking, after the strawberries are soft and juicy and the agar is almost dissolved. This way the blueberries become soft, but retain their round shape and distinct color and flavor.

To prepare pie dough, heat water, oil, and salt together. This mixes the ingredients well, thoroughly dissolves the salt, and makes for smoother dough. Add warmed liquid to flour. Stir to form a kneadable dough, then knead quickly and briefly just enough to make dough smooth. Add more flour only if necessary. Roll dough out immediately as whole wheat pastry flour tends to harden with time and place in oiled pie pan. Crimp edges and bake at 350ºF just until edges are barely golden, about 15 minutes. Allow to cool slightly before filling, or reserve for later use.

Pour filling into prebaked crust. Allow to gel, about three hours at room temperature or less in the refrigerator.

VLF Apple Pie

SERVES 8

> 4 cups apples, shredded or thinly sliced
> 1 6-ounce (170-ml) can frozen apple juice concentrate
> 1 T cornstarch, tapioca or flour
> 1 t vanilla, coriander or fennel or combination

Bring apple juice concentrate to a boil and stir in the thickener which has been blended with a little water. Add the apples, vanilla and spices to the mixture and stir well. Put all into 9-inch pastry shell. If you are going to put on a top crust, moisten the edge of crust and seal together to prevent juice from leaking out. Bake for 45 minutes at 350ºF. May use Fat-Free Pie Crust*.

VLF Fresh Fruit Pie

SERVES 8

> 2 cups cherries or strawberries, fresh or frozen and pitted
> 2 cups fruit juice
> 3 T arrowroot or cornstarch, dissolved in $\frac{1}{4}$ cup water
>   or fruit juice

Fill baked pie shell with fruit mixture. In a saucepan, bring juice to boil. Thicken with arrowroot or cornstarch mixed with water or juice. Cook five minutes. Cool. Pour over fruit. Serve with cashew cream or plain.

VLF Lemon Pie

SERVES 8

> 1$\frac{1}{2}$ cups canned pineapple chunks with juice
> $\frac{3}{4}$ cups dates
> $\frac{1}{2}$ cup cornstarch or arrowroot
> 1 lemon

Blend fruit and thickener until smooth. Cook to thicken. Add finely grated rind of 1 lemon and 2 T juice of fresh lemon.

Pour into pre-baked or no bake pie shell.

TT Carob Mocha Tofu Pie

SERVES 8

Crust:

2 T soy margarine (non-hydrogenated) or unrefined
   coconut butter
1 T cinnamon
1 cup granola

In a saucepan over low heat melt margarine and cinnamon. Stir in granola. Pour into a 9-inch pie pan. (Graham cracker crust is delicious, too.)

Pie:

12 ounces (340 g) tofu, crumbled
1 cup vanilla soy milk (1% or non-fat)
1 T vanilla
¼ cup raw carob powder
¼ cup tahini
¼ cup Sucanat (or turbinado sugar)
2 T grain beverage, coffee or decaf

Blend ingredients until smooth then pour into crust. Chill in refrigerator for several hours.

LF Pumpkin Pie

SERVES 8

1½ cups soy milk (1% or non-fat)
4 T cornstarch
1½ cups cooked pumpkin
½ cup Sucanat (or turbinado sugar) or other
   natural sweetener
½ t salt
1 t cinnamon
½ t ginger
⅛ t cloves

Preheat oven to 375°F. In a large bowl whisk together soy milk and cornstarch until smooth, then blend in remaining ingredients. Pour into an unbaked 9-inch pie shell. Bake in preheated oven for 45 minutes.

LF Raw Nut Fruit Confections

MAKES 6 TO 8 BALLS

Experiment with other nuts or seeds and other dried fruit. These are great for the kids' lunchboxes.

> $^1/_2$ cup raw almonds, ground
> $^1/_4$ cup raisins
> $^1/_4$ cup dates
> 1 t vanilla
> $^1/_2$ banana
> 1 T raw carob powder
> 1 T cinnamon
> coconut, finely shredded (optional)

Process in food processor until a ball forms (May need $^1/_2$ t of water) Break off a golf-ball-size piece and roll it into a ball.

OTHER NUTS:	**OTHER DRIED FRUIT:**
cashews	apricot
peanuts	apples
hazelnuts	peaches
walnuts	papaya

VLF Lo-Fat Oatmeal Date Cookies

MAKES ABOUT 20

Here is a wonderful way to make oatmeal cookies without any added fat.

> $1^1/_2$ cups oats
> 1 t cinnamon
> $^1/_4$ raisins
> $^1/_2$ cup dates
> 1 cup water
> 1 t vanilla
> $^1/_4$ cup maple syrup

Blend $^1/_2$ cup oats until it is a course flour. Mix with the rest of the oats and the other dry ingredients. Blend all wet ingredients and add to dry ingredients. Let sit for 15 minutes. Shape into cookies. Place on non-stick cookie sheet. Bake at 350ºF for 15 minutes.

TT Carob Fudge

SERVES 10

1½ cups carob powder
½ cup sunflower seeds, chopped
½ cup raisins, chopped
½ cup sorghum (or other natural sweetener)
1 cup peanut butter
1½ cups water
1 t vanilla

Combine ingredients and press into shallow rectangular pan. Chill.

LF Caramel Custard (Flan) with Topping

SERVES 9

Flan originated in Spain as a custard with a burnt sugar layer.

Custard:

1 cup water
½ cup plus 1 T agar sea vegetable flakes, well packed
½ cup maple syrup
⅛ cup tahini
¼ t sea salt
3 cups soy milk
1 t vanilla

Caramel Topping:

¼ cup maple syrup
¼ cup water
1 t agar sea vegetable flakes
cinnamon to dust surface

To prepare custard, place all ingredients, except soy milk and vanilla, in pot to soak for five minutes. Bring to boil then simmer until agar completely dissolves, about 10 minutes. Stir with a wire whisk to dissolve tahini. Let cool 3 minutes, then add to soy milk with vanilla. Stir and strain through a fine mesh strainer into 8-inch square 1½-quart baking dish. Let custard set for 15 minutes.

Prepare caramel topping by soaking ingredients, except cinnamon, in small saucepan for 5 minutes then bringing to boil and simmering until agar is dissolved, about 3 minutes. Pour through strainer over custard so a thin layer covers the surface and dust with cinnamon. Allow custard to gel for 2 hours at room temperature, then cut in squares to serve.

LF Millet or Rice Pudding

SERVES 4

Do not forget about this wholesome and tasty dessert.

> 4 cups cooked millet or rice
> 1 cup raisins
> 1/2 cup slivered almonds
> 1 t cinnamon
> 1 t grated orange rind
> 2 1/2-3 cups rice milk or cashew milk
> 1/4 cup maple syrup

Mix together cooked millet or rice and raisins. Put into baking pan and sprinkle with 1/2 cup slivered almonds, cinnamon and grated orange rind. Over this pour the rice milk or cashew milk, mixed with the maple syrup and bake for 3/4 hour. Let cool.

Cashew Milk:

> 1 cup cashews or almonds
> 4 cups water
> 1/2 cup dates
> 1 t vanilla
> pinch of salt

Blend until smooth.

LF Chocolate Pudding

SERVES 3

This is chocolatey satisfying.

> 1 1/2 cups soy milk (1% or non-fat) or rice milk
> 3 T cornstarch
> 1/4 t vanilla
> 1/4 cup maple syrup
> 1/4 cup cocoa powder
> 2 bananas, sliced (optional)

Whisk all the ingredients (except the bananas) together in a pot. Cook over medium heat, stirring constantly, until pudding thickens.

Remove pot from stove. Stir in sliced bananas if desired. Chill for at least 15 minutes before serving.

Variation: Replace chocolate powder with non-dairy carob powder.

VLF Hot Fudge Sundae

SERVES 10

> 2 cups dates
> 2 cups water
> ³/₄ cup carob powder
> 2 t vanilla
> 10 large bananas, frozen and sliced

Heat dates in water and liquefy. Add carob to make dark fudge color. Add vanilla. Pour over frozen sliced bananas and sprinkle with nuts. Note: This can be made by blending the dates in water without heating if the dates are soft. Try adding ¹/₂ cup carob and continue adding to taste. You may like less than ³/₄ cup carob.

VLF Berry Sherbet

SERVES 4

> 1 pint berries, frozen
> ¹/₂ cup pineapple juice
> 1 banana, frozen

Blend until smooth. Serve

LF Ginger Crinkle Cookies

MAKES 2¹/₂ DOZEN

> ¹/₃ cup macadamia, cashew or almond butter
> ³/₄ cup Sucanat (or turbinado sugar) or sweetener
> ¹/₄ cup molasses
> 3 T water
> 2 cups flour
> 2 t baking powder
> ¹/₂ t salt
> 2 t ginger
> 2 t cinnamon

Cream nut butter and sugar, add molasses and water. Beat until smooth.

Stir together the dry ingredients, then gradually add them to the butter mixture. Mix thoroughly.

Roll dough into balls the size of walnuts, then place on an greased cookie sheet about 2 inches apart. Bake at 350ºF for 8-10 minutes until golden brown on bottoms and edges.

TT Pecan Drops

MAKES 30

These are delicious and easy to make.

>1 cup pitted moist dates
>2 cups pecans, finely ground
>1 t orange zest (finely grated orange peel)
>30 pecan halves

Chop the dates coarsely, then add the ground pecans and orange zest, kneading together with you hands to form a dough. Roll dough into balls the size of walnuts and place on an ungreased baking sheet. They will not spread, so they can be placed close together. Press a pecan half into the center of each.

Bake in the upper third of a 325ºF preheated oven for 12-15 minutes, or until bottoms are lightly browned

LF Apple Cranberry Crisp

SERVES 8 TO 10

>1 12-ounce (340 g) package of cranberries or
> about 3 cups
>2 large tart apples, cored and sliced
>1/2 cup Sucanat (or turbinado sugar) or other
> natural sweetener
>1 T flour
>1 t cinnamon
>1 1/2 cups rolled oats
>1/3 cup whole-wheat flour
>4 T Sucanat (or turbinado sugar) or other
> natural sweetener
>1/3 cup plain or vanilla soy yogurt

Preheat over to 350ºF.

Rinse the cranberries. In a mixing bowl, combine the cranberries, apples, sugar, flour and cinnamon. Stir together, then transfer to a 9x13-inch baking dish.

In the same mixing bowl, stir together the rolled oats and remaining ingredients, until the texture is uniformly crumbly. Sprinkle evenly over fruit.

Bake at 350ºF for 45 minutes, until lightly browned. Let stand 10 minutes before serving.

136

VLF Baked Apples

SERVES 4

Simple, yet delicious.

> 4 large, tart apples
> 3-5 pitted dates, chopped
> 1 t cinnamon

Wash apples, then remove core to within ¼ inch of bottoms. Combine dates and cinnamon, then distribute equally into the centers of the apples. Place in a baking dish filled with ¼ inch of hot water, and bake at 350ºF for 40-60 minutes. Serve hot or chilled.

Serving Suggestion: Top with a dollop of almond or cashew cream recipe below.

TT Almond or Cashew Cream

MAKES 1 CUP

> ½ cup blanched almonds or cashews
> ½-¾ cup cold water
> 6-8 dates, pitted
> 1 t vanilla
> 1 banana

Grind the nuts in a blender first. Add all ingredients and blend. Chill.

VLF Pears in Apple/Orange Sauce

MAKES 4 SERVINGS

> ⅔ cup apple juice
> 1 t fresh orange peel, grated
> 1 t vanilla extract
> 2 t Sucanat (or turbinado sugar)
> 4 small pears, peeled, cored and sliced into ⅛ inch slices

In a large non-stick skillet, combine apple juice, orange peel, vanilla and sugar. Add pears.

Bring to a boil over medium heat, stirring frequently. Cover and simmer 5 minutes, or until pears are just tender, stirring several times.

Serve warm or cold.

LF Fruit Bars

SERVES 10 TO 12

> 2 cups brown rice, cooked
> 1 banana
> 1 cup raisins
> 1 cup dates, chopped
> 1/2 cup whole-wheat flour
> 1 1/2 cups water
> 1/4 cup maple syrup
> 1 t salt
> 1 T cinnamon
> 2 t lemon extract
> 1 t vanilla
> 4 cups granola

Blend brown rice in as small amount of the water as possible. Blend in the banana then add the raisins and dates and blend until smooth adding the balance of the water as you blend. Do not add more water, but stop blender and push mixture with spoon until it will blend. Pour into large bowl and add all of the ingredients except the granola.

Place granola in plastic bag and roll with rolling pin until medium course then add to mixture. Pour into a 9x13 pan, which as been oiled and then dusted lightly with whole-wheat flour and then bake at 400ºF degrees for 15 minutes or until fork comes out clean.

TT Gandhi Good Bars

SERVES 10

> 1 cup peanut butter
> 1 cup organic brown rice syrup
> 1 t unrefined almond oil
> 1 cup puffed rice
> 1 cup puffed millet
> 1/2 cup granola
> 1/2 cup shredded coconut
> 1/4 cup carob date chips

Melt peanut butter and rice syrup together over low heat.

Gradually stir in remaining ingredients. Put into a 9x13 pan lightly greased with almond oil.

Refrigerate. Cut into squares.

Enjoy a variety of Gandhi goodness by mixing and matching proportions of nut butters in place of peanut butter. Almond butter is always a favorite. Or try ½ cup rice syrup with ½ cup maple syrup. If you do not have millet, use all puffed rice. Look for the wide range of carob chips at health food stores. Experiment.

TT Carrot Cake

SERVES 12

> 2 cups carrots, grated
> 1½ cups raisins
> 2 cups water
> ½ cup unrefined almond or melted coconut oil
> 1¼ cups maple syrup
> 1½ t cinnamon
> 1½ t allspice
> ½ t cloves
> 1½ t salt
> 3 cups unbleached or whole-wheat pastry flour
> 1½ t baking soda
> 1 t black walnut extract

Simmer grated carrots, raisins and water in a saucepan for 10 minutes. Add oil, maple syrup, cinnamon, allspice, cloves, salt and walnut extract and allow to stand until cool.

Stir together the flour and soda, then add to the cooled carrots and stir just to moisten all ingredients. Bake at 350°F in a greased 9x9-inch pan (or a tube pan or 2 loaf pans) until toothpick inserted into the center comes out clean, 45 minutes to 1 hour. Frost with Tofu Cream Frosting when completely cooled.

Tofu Cream Frosting

It is important that the tofu, which is the basis of this frosting, be fresh. Fresh tofu has a neutral or slightly sweet taste. As it gets older, it develops a sourness that is not appropriate in frosting.

> 1 cup fresh tofu
> 1 T oil
> 2 T fresh lemon juice
> 3-4 T maple syrup
> ¼ t salt
> ½ t vanilla

Combine ingredients in a blender and blend until very smooth. Scrape sides of blender often with a rubber spatula, pushing the tofu towards the center of the blender. Makes enough to generously frost on 9x9-inch cake.

ᴛᴛ Chocolate Cake

MAKES 12 SERVINGS

Cake:
- ³/₄ cup whole-wheat flour
- ²/₃ cup oat bran or 3 ounces
- ¹/₄ cup cocoa, unsweetened
- 1 t baking powder
- 1 t baking soda
- 3 T flax seeds, ground then blended with ¹/₄ cup water
- ¹/₂ cup applesauce, unsweetened
- ²/₃ cup apple juice
- 2 t vanilla extract
- ¹/₄ t almond extract

Topping:
- 2 T walnuts, chopped or ¹/₂ ounce
- 2 T chocolate or carob chips

Preheat oven to 325°F.

Lightly oil an 8-inch square baking pan.

In a large bowl, combine flour, oat bran, cocoa, baking powder and baking soda. Mix well.

In another bowl combine remaining cake ingredients. Beat with a fork or wire whisk until blended. Add to dry mixture, mixing until all ingredients are moistened.

Place in prepared pan. Sprinkle nuts and chocolate or carob chips evenly over cake, pressing them lightly into the cake.

Bake 35 minutes until a toothpick inserted in the center of the cake comes out clean. Cool in pan on wire rack. Cut into squares to serve.

Milks and Creams

Try out the soy and rice milks in the natural food stores and find the one you like. Use it as you would have used dairy milk. These store in your pantry for a long time until you open the package but then you must refrigerate the milk. At that point, it'll stay fresh for about 8 days.

The nut creams are rich and delicious. Use them as toppings for cooked or baked fruit, for fruitcrisps, for rice or millet pudding, on a bowl of fruit salad or on pies. Just try not to get addicted!

VLF Basic Rice Milk

MAKES ABOUT 3½ CUPS

Good for general cooking

> 2 cups brown rice, cooked very well
> 2 cups hot water

Place rice and water alternately in blender and blend until smooth. This will be quite thick and gets even thicker as it sets. It may be used in gravies, sauces and soups in place of milk.

LF Almond Milk

MAKES 2 CUPS

> ½ cup raw almonds
> 2 cups water
> 2 dates

Blend raw almonds first into a powder. Add water and dates. Liquefy. Strain.

VLF Banana Milk

MAKES 3 CUPS

> 2 cups ice cold water
> 2 ripe bananas
> ½ T vanilla
> 1 T maple syrup

Blend well and pour on cereal.

TT Sunny Milk

MAKES 5 CUPS

> $^{1}/_{2}$ cup raw sunflower seeds
> 1 cup ice cold water
> 4 cups ice cold water
> 1 T vanilla
> 2 T maple syrup

Blend seeds and 1 cup cold water until smooth. Add 4 cups cold water and the rest of the ingredients. Blend to mix.

Serve over cereal.

TT Cashew Cream

MAKES 1 CUP

> 1 cup white grape juice
> $^{1}/_{2}$ cup cashew nuts
> $^{1}/_{4}$ t vanilla

Blend until smooth and creamy. Serve as topping for fruit pie or puddings.

LF Strawberry Cream

MAKES 3 CUPS

> 1$^{1}/_{2}$ cup water (cold)
> $^{1}/_{2}$ cup cashews
> $^{1}/_{2}$ cup cooked rice
> 1 cup frozen strawberries
> $^{1}/_{4}$ cup dates
> pinch of salt
> 1 t lemon juice

Blend. Chill until served.

Variations: Use any other frozen fruit in place of strawberries.

142

Beverages and Snacks

Delicious smoothies and shakes can be made easily and quickly. Frozen bananas are the key to a great smoothie or shake. Let bananas ripen until they have brown spots. Peel the bananas and place in baggies in the freezer. These stay for at least two months and can be used as needed.

Use the frozen banana as your base, and experiment with different fruit juices, fruits and nuts or nutmilks. It is a wonderful beverage and snack for a youngster home from school and hungry.

The snack recipes are low-fat, and tasty treats.

LF The Best Date Shake in the World

SERVES 2

> 1¹/₂ cups Almond Milk*
> 2 frozen bananas
> 6 large seedless dates, fresh or frozen

Place milk and fruit in a blender. Blend until thick and creamy. If you like a thinner shake use 1¹/₂ bananas.

TT Banini (Vanilla Malted)

SERVES 4

> 3 cups water (ice cold)
> 4 bananas, frozen and sliced
> 1 ripe banana, sliced
> ¹/₄ cup tahini
> 2 T sweetener
> 1 t vanilla

Combine all the ingredients in a blender; blend at medium speed until creamy. If you use a food processor, you can omit the liquid. Chill in freezer.

LF Fruit Whiz

SERVES 2

> 1 cup soy milk, low-fat
> 1 t vanilla extract
> 2 large oranges, peeled and sectioned

1 large banana, peeled
5 ice cubes

Place all the ingredients in a blender and blend until smooth. Serve immediately.

Variation: Substitute peeled tangerines for the oranges. Make sure to remove all seeds before blending.

VLF Mochi Puffs

SERVES 3 TO 4

Mochi are wonderful chewy rice cakes. Usually found in the frozen section of the natural food store, when baked, they puff up into fragrant, satisfying morsels. Look for a mochi in a variety of flavors besides natural, such as cinnamon, sesame or garlic.

1 pack mochi
salsa

Preheat oven to 450°F. Break apart mochi, place on top rack of oven, bake until toasty, approximately 5-10 minutes. Arrange on a serving platter serve with salsa in center.

VLF Lo-Cal Popcorn

Mix air-popped popcorn with nutritional yeast, aminos, cayenne, lemon juice and whatever spices delight you – curry is great!

VLF Popcorn Treat

popcorn
nutritional yeast
water
Bragg Liquid Aminos

Pop popcorn in an air popper until done. Cut the strength of the Bragg Liquid Aminos by combining ½ water and ½ Aminos in a spray bottle. Spray popcorn with mixture and sprinkle with nutritional yeast.

TT Mini Pizzas

SERVES 2 TO 3

1 stalk broccoli, chopped
2 celery stalks, chopped finely

1 onion, minced
$\frac{1}{2}$ t oregano
1 garlic clove, minced
2 T unrefined oil
1 15-ounce (425-ml) can tomato sauce
3 English muffins containing no animal products

Sauté broccoli, celery, onion, oregano and garlic in oil over medium-high heat for 5 minutes, until broccoli is tender, yet firm.

Add tomato sauce and continue heating for 3 minutes longer. Remove from heat.

Split English muffins in half. Spoon sauce over muffins. Sprinkle with nutritional yeast if desired.

VLF No-Oil Chips and Quick Salsa*

1 dozen corn tortillas
1 recipe Quick Salsa*

Toast whole tortillas on oven rack for 10-15 minutes until crisp (who needs all that oil?). Break apart into quarters and serve around a center bowl of salsa.

LF Tofu Yogurt

SERVES 2 TO 4

1 cake tofu or 8 ounces (227 g) (fat-reduced)
1 banana, frozen and sliced
1 ripe banana, sliced
2 T sweetener
$\frac{1}{4}$ cup fruit juice
1 t vanilla
1 cup strawberries or 1 cup blueberries

Combine all the ingredients in a blender; blend at medium speed until creamy. If you use a food processor – you can omit the liquid. Chill in freezer.

LF Pita Chips

SERVES 8

3 pita breads
2 t extra virgin olive oil

* Recipe in Recipe Collection

145

$^1\!/_2$ t paprika
1$^1\!/_2$ small garlic cloves, minced
1 t oregano
$^1\!/_2$ t salt (optional)

Split pita breads in half. Cut each half into several 2-inch triangles.

Place the cut bread on a lightly oiled cookie sheet. Sprinkle bread with half the oil, and half the paprika, garlic, oregano, and if you like, salt.

Place the bread under a broiler until it begins to brown. Turn the bread over and sprinkle with remaining oil and spices. Place the bread back under the broiler for 2 minutes longer. remove the chips. Once the chips cool they will be crisp and delicious.

Thanksgiving

A warm, loving time of year, when friends and family come together and share friendship, love and good food. There is nothing quite like the feeling of preparing a feast that everyone fully enjoys and knowing that the food served is also nourishing and unharmful – after all, these are your loved ones.

The most important thing to remember is the spirit in which the food is made and the beautiful way in which it is served.

The visual is very important. Try some of these recipes at your next Thanksgiving.

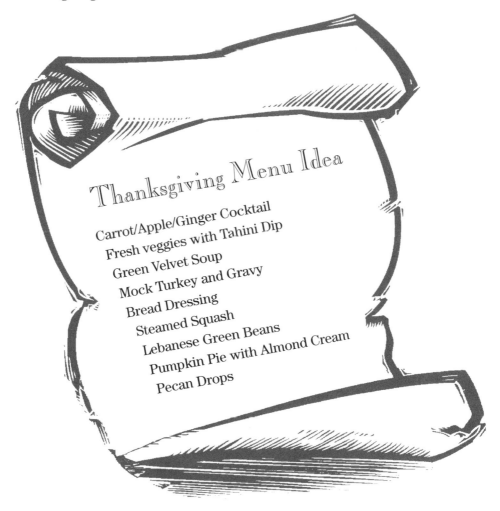

Thanksgiving Menu Idea

Carrot/Apple/Ginger Cocktail
Fresh veggies with Tahini Dip
Green Velvet Soup
Mock Turkey and Gravy
Bread Dressing
Steamed Squash
Lebanese Green Beans
Pumpkin Pie with Almond Cream
Pecan Drops

TT Mock Turkey with Gravy

SERVES 4

Mock Turkey:
> 8 ounces (227-ml) tofu, well-drained
> ½ cup natural soy sauce

Place tofu in a bowl with soy sauce and let sit a few minutes on each side to soak up soy sauce and turn brown. Place on top of steamer rack with small amount of water and steam with cover 20 minutes.

When tofu is done, remove from steamer. Slice in ¼-½-inch slices. Place in a baking pan, top with gravy and broil in oven a few minutes. Tofu can also be fried in a little extra virgin olive oil before topping with gravy. Serve with Basic Vegetarian Gravy* (Choose your favorite variation.)

TT Thanksgiving Chestnut Croquettes

SERVES 12 TO 14

> 4 T oil
> 1 cup celery stalks and leaves, chopped
> ½ cup onion, minced
> 4 cups steamed brown rice
> 2 cups boiled chestnuts or chickpeas (garbanzo beans),
>   finely chopped
> ½ cup parsley, minced
> ¼ cup almond butter or peanut butter
> 1 t sage
> 1 t "Chicken" Style Seasoning* (recipe at the end of
>   this section)
> ¼ t thyme
> salt to taste
> bread crumbs
> oil
> paprika

In a skillet heat oil, celery and onion. Sauté just until golden yellow. Add some bread crumbs (about ¼ cup). Heat, stirring to prevent excessive browning. Turn into a deep bowl. Add remaining ingredients except bread crumbs, oil and paprika, mixing well with hands or spoon.

Add soft bread crumbs as necessary to make desired consistency for shaping croquettes. Shape croquettes and sprinkle with oil and paprika. Bake on cookie sheet or pan fry in a little olive oil until golden brown.

* Recipe in Recipe Collection

148

TT Rice Dressing

SERVES 6 TO 8

This dressing is made with a combination of wild rice and brown rice. You could also substitute some of the specialty rices, such as Wehani or Basmati for part of the brown rice.

3 cups water
$1/4$ t salt
$3/4$ cup long grain brown rice
$3/4$ cup wild rice
2 T extra virgin olive oil
1 small onion, chopped
1 pound (454 g) mushrooms, cleaned and sliced
$1/2$ cup parsley, finely chopped
1 cup celery, sliced
$1/2$ t salt
$1/4$ t sage
$1/8$ t each black pepper, marjoram, thyme
$1/2$ cup pecan halves, broken lengthwise

Bring water to boil and add salt and rice. Lower to simmer, then cover and cook until all water is absorbed, about 50 minutes.

In a large ovenproof skillet, melt the oil and sauté the onion and mushrooms until the onion is transparent. Add the parsley, celery, cooked rice, seasonings, and pecans. Stir to mix, then cover and bake at 350°F for 15 minutes.

LF Bread Dressing

SERVES 8

1 small onion, chopped
2 T extra virgin olive oil
3 cups mushrooms, sliced
1 cup celery, sliced
4 cups cubed bread
$1/4$ cup fresh parsley, finely chopped
$1/4$ t sage and thyme
$1/8$ t marjoram and black pepper
$1/2$ t salt
1 cup (approximately) very hot water or vegetable stock

149

In a large kettle or skillet, heat oil and sauté onion for 5 minutes then add sliced mushrooms and celery. Cover and cook over medium heat until mushrooms are brown, then add the bread and seasonings. Stir in water or stock, a little at a time until dressing obtains desired moistness.

Place in a non-stick 1-quart baking dish, cover and bake for 20 minutes at 350ºF. Remove cover and bake 10 minutes longer.

LF Thanksgiving Stuffing

SERVES 8

2 cups whole-wheat or other whole grain bread crumbs
$\frac{1}{2}$ cup lentils, cooked
$\frac{1}{2}$ cup walnuts, finely chopped
2-3 T extra virgin olive oil
2 garlic cloves
1 onion, chopped
$\frac{1}{2}$ cup celery
$\frac{1}{2}$ cup tomatoes, blended and strained
1 t sage, finely crushed
$\frac{1}{2}$ t thyme
$\frac{1}{2}$ t vegetable salt
$\frac{1}{2}$ cup black olives, chopped
2 T arrowroot mixed in 4 T water

Combine first 3 ingredients and set aside. Sauté next 4 ingredients together in a skillet. Add next 4 ingredients and cook for about 5 minutes. Add the last 2 ingredients. Stir in well, then pour into mixture of dry ingredients.

Place in oiled loaf pan and bake at 350ºF for 1 hour. Baste the top every 15 minutes with melted butter. Good served with Mock Turkey and Gravy*.

VLF Thanksgiving Cranberry Sauce

SERVES 8

4 cups cranberries
2 cups water
$1\frac{1}{2}$ cups maple syrup
1 T orange zest

Cook cranberries in water until they start popping. Press through a coarse sieve. Add maple syrup and orange zest. Simmer 2 minutes.

* Recipe in Recipe Collection

VLF "Chicken" Style Seasoning

MAKES 1¼ CUPS

> 1 cup nutritional yeast
> 2½ t sweet pepper flakes, powdered
> 3 t onion powder
> 3½ t salt
> 2½ t sage
> 2½ t thyme
> 4 garlic cloves, minced
> 1¼ t marjoram
> 1¼ t rosemary

Mix. Omit or add ingredients as you desire. Store in a container tightly closed.

VLF Carrot-Apple-Ginger Cocktail

SERVES 4

This recipe is great for an afternoon pick-me-up and a delicious way to start any meal. A juicer is required. I highly suggest that, especially for juicing, you use organic produce.

> 12 medium carrots, 1 apple, ½-inch piece of fresh ginger, peeled

Cut all ingredients into the size that will fit into your juicer. Juice all ingredients. Stir and serve as soon as possible. Enjoy!

Thanksgiving Suggestions:

Other recipes in this book that lend themselves beautifully to Thanksgiving feasts for the eye and palate.

Jeff's Favorite "Neat" Loaf with Country Gravy	Broccoli Italiano
	Tofu Cornbread
Tofu Loaf with Country Gravy	Mashed Potatoes and Gravy
Millet Mashed Potatoes with Country Gravy	Brown or Chicken-Like Gravy
	Fat-Free Gravy
Corn Chowder	Apple Pie
Lebanese Green Beans	Apple-Cranberry Crisp
Vegetables with Dill	Pears in Apple/Orange Sauce
Sesame Carrots with Dill Weed	

Glossary of Terms

Arrowroot: a white powder used as a thickening agent instead of cornstarch or kuzu. It can also be used as a binder in egg-free baking.

Breads: an excellent source of protein and fiber and can be used at almost every meal. "Pocket" pita breads, dark Essene breads, whole-grain rye bread, "multi-grain" breads are all delicious. Read labels and avoid white breads and those containing eggs, milk, whey or honey. Rye breads are often made without dairy products.

Bragg Liquid Aminos: a wonderful soy sauce-like substance made by extracting amino acids from organic soy beans. Ideal for those who suffer from yeast sensitivities as its is not fermented. Use instead of soy sauce or tamari.

Carob: looks like cocoa powder but it is not. Carob has its own unique, sweet taste, but can be used in the same ways you would use cocoa powder. It is much more nutritious than chocolate and contains none of the caffeine-like stimulants.

Flaxseed Oil: a nutritional oil, rich in essential fats, found in the refrigerator of natural food stores. Take 1 tablespoon daily for dry skin to dandruff. *Do not cook* with flaxseed oil as it breaks down with heat. It can be brushed on bread, poured over vegetables or mixed in salad dressings.

Flax Seeds: an excellent source of essential fatty acids, linoleic acid and also dietary fiber. Use in baking as an egg substitute. To substitute for 1 egg blend 1 T flax seeds and 1/4 cup water in a blender for 1 to 2 minutes until the mixture is thick and has the consistency of beaten egg whites. Fold into the other ingredients.

Kuzu (or kudzu): a white, lumpy substance resembling chalk, extracted from the large root of the kuzu vine. It serves as a thickener to help create smooth sauces, soups and desserts. Sold in natural food stores and Asian markets.

Legumes: protein bonanzas! Anything that grows in a pod. Of best use to the body when eaten with whole grains: 2 1/2 parts grain to 1 part legumes. Beans of all types: lentils, chickpeas (garbanzo beans), peas, bean sprouts, tofu and other soy products. Use in soups, stews, tacos, chili, casseroles and mash into sandwich spreads.

Mirin: found in most natural food stores or supermarkets, this is a sweet, low-alcohol japanese cooking wine.

Miso (ME-so): (Asian) a thick paste made from cooked soybeans (and optionally rice or other grains) that are aged with salt from two months to several years. Primarily used to flavor soups and broths, miso is rich in enzymes and known for its beneficial effect on digestion. In general, the longer it is aged the darker its color and the stronger (saltier) its flavor.

Nutritional Yeast: pleasant yellow flakes with delicious cheesy taste; great on salads, in soups and sprinkled on casseroles. Often fortified with vitamin B-12; check label to be sure it contains at least 1 microgram of vitamin B-12 per tablespoon.

Organic: grown and processed without chemical fertilizers, insecticides or additives. Look for official verification on the label. For example, "Organically grown in accordance with Section 26569.11, California Health and Safety Code." Best if locally-grown.

Pastas: noodles of all types add substance to Oriental and Italian entrées and are available in many different styles such as artichoke spaghetti, vegetable spirals. They are a convenient base from which to plan a dinner.

Rice Dream: low fat, non dairy beverage made from organic brown rice. It has a hint of natural sweetness from the rice for use in savory recipes (soups, sauces, casseroles) diluted approximately 3 to 4 parts Rice Dream to 1 part water. Natural food stores often carry delicious Rice Dream frozen desserts in the freezer case.

Sea Vegetables: kelp, dulse, nori, kombu, arame. These contain trace minerals like iodine, manganese, selenium and calcium. They are good on salads, in soups and in dressings.

Seeds: high in protein and essential oils. For example, sunflower, sesame, pumpkin. Purchase raw. Roast in the oven for topping and treats. Blend with cold water and a dash of sweetener to make a milk for pouring over cereal, baking and so on. Store in clean, dry covered containers in refrigerator.

Seitan (SAY-tan): wheat gluten, also known as "wheat meat" in North America, is found in the refrigerator case in natural food stores. This high protein, low-fat meat substitute developed long ago in the Orient is now becoming popular in vegetarian cooking in this country. It is a refined product since most of the starch and bran are removed from the gluten dough but because of its meaty texture and good taste it is useful as a transitional food to substitute for red meat.

Shoyu (SHOW-you): naturally brewed soy sauce made from soybeans, wheat, water and sea salt. It is processed in the traditional Japanese way and aged for two to three years. No coloring or preservatives are used. Found in natural food stores (most supermarket soy sauce is highly processed).

Soy Milk: non-dairy beverage derived from soybeans typically sold in vacuum packed boxes, dated, with a shelf life of several months. It is an excellent milk substitute for cooking, baking, sauces, on cereal or as beverage. There are several different brands with different ingredients and tastes. Also different flavors such as plain (for cooking) or vanilla and carob (sweeter for beverage or cereal). Read labels to compare fat content, calories and nutrients; also, some brands use organic ingredients. Look for fortified soy milk that compares to the nutrient content in cows milk.

Sprouts: high in protein and vitamins. For example, alfalfa, lentils, mung beans. Easy to grow yourself or buy fresh at the supermarket.

Super Blue-Green Algae: this dried powder product is one of the best sources of plant protein, minerals, chlorophyll and vitamin B-12. A nutritious addition to smoothies or health drinks. (See resources for distributor)

Sweeteners: sorghum, maple syrup, barley malt syrup, rice syrup, natural fruits, fruit juices, dates, puréed fruits in baked goods. Use these to replace honey and sugar.

Tahini (tah-HEE-nee): paste of ground raw or roasted sesame seeds also called sesame butter. Rich in calcium.

Tamari (tah-MAH-ree): natural soy sauce primarily made from soybeans, with up to 10% wheat. Also available wheat free with a slightly stronger flavor than shoyu.

Tempeh (TEM-pay): a cultured soyfood, high in protein originally developed by Indonesians. A sliceable cake of soybeans that have been cooked and split to remove the hull. A culture is added to the cooked soybeans and they are allowed to age for one to two days. The culture covers the cake holding it together. Tempeh has a distinctive aroma, flavor, and texture. It can be sliced thin and fried, braised, boiled or baked. Often a good meat substitute in stews and casseroles.

Tofu (TOW-foo): high-protein pressed curd of soybean milk, also called "bean curd", originating in China and Japan. Mild tasting, it readily absorbs seasoning when marinated, baked, boiled or fried. It is also a good egg substitute in baking: to replace one egg use 1/4 cup soft tofu blended until smooth in a blender. Buy calcium-precipitated tofu.

TVP: (Texturized Vegetable Protein): granules made from soybeans; prepared by adding hot water. Adds a hearty "ground beef" texture to spaghetti sauce, chili, soups, casseroles and burgers. TVP is usually fortified with vitamin B-12.

Vegetarian Broth Powder: this powder, made from a combination of spices and herbs, can be found in the spice section of a natural food store. Although vegetarian based, these broth powders come in various flavors such as chicken or beef. Excellent for flavoring soups, sauces, dressings or stir-fries.

Yellow Vegetables: high in vitamin A and beta carotene. Use in such dishes as vegetable bakes, steamed in side dishes or soups. For example, carrots, sweet potato, squash (summer, spaghetti, butternut, hubbard, acorn, etc.) parsnips, rutabaga and pumpkin.

Recipe Index

157

Resources

The books and organizations below will help you further your journey to better health. You will find you are far from alone on this journey and that there is a wealth of information and people to assist you.

Recommended Reading

The Power of Your Plate ....by Neal Barnard, MD
Foods That Cause You to Lose Weight .....by Neal Barnard, MD
A Vegetarian Primer ....by Peter Burwash
Ageless Body, Timeless Mind ....by Deepak Chopra
The American Vegetarian Cookbook ....by Marilyn Diamond
The Almost No Fat Cookbook ....by Bryanna Clark Grogan
Vegan Nutrition: Pure & Simple ....by Michael Klaper, MD
Pregnancy, Children & the Vegan Diet ..by Michael Klaper, MD
The Menopause Self Help Book ....by Susan M. Lark, MD
PMS Self-Help Book: A Woman's Guide ..by Susan M. Lark, MD
American Macrobiotic Kitchen ....by Meredith McCarty
Fresh from a Vegetarian Kitchen ....by Meredith McCarty
*McDougall's Medicine: A Challenging
Second Opinion* ....by John McDougall, MD
Becoming Vegetarian ....by Vesanto Melina, RD
The Love Powered Diet ....by Victoria Moran
Encyclopedia of Natural Medicine ....by Michael Murray
*Dr. Dean Ornish's Program for
Reversing Heart Disease* ....by Dean Ornish, MD
Stress, Diet and Your Heart ....by Dean Ornish, MD
Do Not Drink Your Milk! ....by Frank A. Oski, MD
The Peaceful Palate ....by Jennifer Raymond
Diet for a New America ....by John Robbins
Return to the Joy of Health ....by Zoltan Rona, MD
The Canadian Vegetarian Dining Guide ...by Lynne Tomlinson
Fresh Vegetables and Fruit Juices ....by Norman Walker
Simply Vegan ....by Debra Wasserman
Reversing Diabetes ....by Julian Whitaker, MD

Periodicals

Living Health PO Box 6769 Syracuse NY

Nutrition Action Center for Science in the Public Interest
1501 – 16th St NW Washington DC 20036

Veggie Life PO Box 412 Mt. Morris IL 61054-8163

Vegetarian Times PO Box 446 Mt. Morris IL 61054

National Organizations

Alive Academy of Nutrition
7436 Fraser Park Drive, Burnaby
BC V5J 5B9
604-435-1919
*Offers a wide variety of
homeopathic and natural diet
home study courses as well as the*
Vancouver Vegetarian Education
Exchange. *This group meets to
share recipes and discuss the
growth and development of
Vancouver's vegetarian
community.*

**American Natural Hygiene
Society**
PO Box 30630
Tampa FL 33630
813-855-6607

**Canadian Natural Health
Association**
5 - 439 Wellington Street West
Toronto ON M5V 1E7
416-977-2642

American Vegan Society
501 Old Harding Hwy
Malaga, NJ 08328
*This organization has a
newsletter and carries many
cookbooks, videos and audio
cassettes on the vegan lifestyle.*

Toronto Vegetarian Association
736 Bathurst Street
Toronto ON M5S 2R4
416-533-3897
Publishes Toronto's Lifelines
*newsletter to improve awareness
and aid Toronto's growing
vegetarian community.*

EarthSave Canada
Vancouver BC
604-731-5885
*A dedicated organization based
on John Robbins' book* A Diet for a
New America.

Earthsave USA
709 Frederick Street
Santa Cruz CA 95062
408-423-4069
*Healthy school lunch program –
effective tool for introducing
health supporting food into
schools.*

Institute of Nutrition Education
342 - 1601 North Sepulveda
Boulevard
Manhattan Beach CA 90266
310-374-3733
*Nutrition education and
information for health
professionals.*

North American Vegetarian Society

PO Box 72
Dolgeville NY 13329
518-568-7970
Membership organization, publishes quarterly Vegetarian Voice *newsletter. Sponsors conferences; mail-order source for books, tapes, and videos. Vegetarian Express Fast Food Campaign project encourages major chains to offer low-fat vegan entrées.*

Physician's Committee For Responsible Medicine

PO Box 6322
Washington DC 20015
Headed by Neal Barnard, MD. Has a monthly newsletter and a nutrition program for corporations or speakers.

Vegetarian Education Network

c/o Sally Clinton
PO Box 3347
West Chester, PA 19380
215-696-VNET
Promotes meatless school lunches.

Vegetarian Resource Group

PO Box 1463
Baltimore, MD 21203
301-366-8343
Membership group, publishes bimonthly Vegetarian Journal *with articles on nutrition, recipes, and information on regional groups. Produces educational materials including books, a color poster and a packet of "quantity" recipes for institutional cooks*

For Super Blue-Green Algae products contact Paulette Eisen at,

1824 Hillhurst Avenue
Los Angelos CA 90027
310-289-4173

A Diet for All Reasons Products

A Diet for All Reasons - Nutrition Guide & Recipe Book

Compiled by Paulette Eisen as a companion to the video below, this cookbook offers advice and guidelines to anyone wanting to change to a healthy vegan diet. This well organized cholesterol-free cookbook offers over 150 exciting recipes in a wide range of tasty meals and snacks.

A Diet for All Reasons Video

In this powerful one-hour presentation, Dr. Klaper clearly demonstrates how and why the foods we eat can either support our health or contribute to disease. This convincing evidence will change the way you think about food. It is also available in the European PAL format.

A Diet for All Reasons Wellness Series

Consists of seven audiotapes by Dr. Klaper in a vinyl album and includes a laminated nutrition chart. These informative and entertaining tapes deal with many of today's most important health issues. The library consists of the following seven tapes:

1. Weight Loss I & II
2. Diabetes, Hypoglycemia and Cancer
3. Healthy Pregnancy and Raising Healthy Children
4. Osteoporosis and Sex & Impotence
5. Exercise and Stress Management
6. Arthritis and Allergies & Auto-immune Diseases
7. Heart Disease & Healthy Arteries I & II

For more information contact:

Paulette Eisen   *OR*
1824 Hillhurst Avenue
Los Angeles CA 90027 USA
310-389-4173

Alive Books
Burnaby BC V5H 3X1 Canada
800-661-0303

Academy of Nutrition | *offers a series of homestudy courses including* Vegetarianism – *The Diet for All Reasons*

Which is an elective for the Nutritional Consulting Diploma and offers students the opportunity to study and understand the healthy alternative of vegetarianism. Throughout the 12 lessons, students will enjoy learning the 'ins and outs' of raw food values, protein, vegetarian kitchens and the transition to a vegetarian diet. The price of this home study course includes the above books and tapes as supplemental study materials. Students will receive an appropriate credit if they are already in possession of this material.

For more information contact: **Alive Academy of Nutrition**
7436 Fraser Park Drive, Burnaby BC V5J 5B9 Phone: 604-435-1919

Other titles by Alive Books

Return to the Joy of Health
Natural medicine and alternative treatments for all your health complaints.
Dr. Zoltan Rona, 408 pp softcover

Fats That Heal Fats That Kill
The complete guide to fats, oils, cholesterol and human health.
Udo Erasmus, 480 pp softcover

Allergies: Disease in Disguise
How to heal your allergic condition permanently and naturally.
Carolee Bateson-Koch DC ND, 224 pp softcover

The Breuss Cancer Cure
Advice for prevention and natural treatment of cancer, leukemia and other seemingly incurable diseases.
Rudolf Breuss (Translated from German), 112 pp softcover

Healing with Herbal Juices
A practical guide to herbal juice therapy: nature's preventative medicine.
Siegfried Gursche, 240 pp softcover

Kombucha Rediscovered!
A Guide to the Medicinal Benefits of an Ancient Healing Tea
Klaus Kaufmann, 96 pp softcover

Silica – The Forgotten Nutrient
Healthy skin, shiny hair, strong bones, beautiful nails. A guide to the vital role of organic vegetal silica in nutrition, health, longevity and medicine.
Klaus Kaufmann, 128 pp softcover

Silica – The Amazing Gel
An essential mineral for radiant health, recovery and rejuvenation.
Klaus Kaufmann, 176 pp softcover

The Joy of Juice Fasting
For health, cleansing and weight loss.
Klaus Kaufmann, 114 pp softcover

Devil's Claw Root and Other Natural Remedies for Arthritis
A herbal remedy has helped free thousands of arthritis sufferers from crippling pain.
Rachel Carston (Revised by Klaus Kaufmann), 128 pp softcover

Making Sauerkraut and Pickled Vegetables at Home
The original lactic acid fermentation method.
Annelies Schoeneck, 80 pp softcover

International Health News Yearbook (Annual)
The latest, most important discoveries in nutrition, health and medicine.
Hans Larsen, 96 pp softcover

All books are available at your local health food store or from
***alive* books**, PO Box 80055, Burnaby BC V5H 3X1